101 Pearls

in
Refractive, Cataract, and Corneal Surgery

SECOND EDITION

Edited by

Samir A. Melki, MD, PhD
Director and Founder, Boston Eye Group
Clinical Instructor, Harvard Medical School
Boston, Massachusetts

and

Dimitri T. Azar, MD
Professor, Field Chair and Head
Department of Ophthalmology and Visual Science
University of Illinois Eye Center
Chicago, Illinois

SLACK
INCORPORATED

Delivering the best in health care information and education worldwide www.slackbooks.com

ISBN-10: 1-55642-684-4
ISBN-13: 978-1-55642-684-1

Copyright © 2006 by SLACK Incorporated

The procedures and practices described in this book should be implemented in a manner consistent with the professional standards set for the circumstances that apply in each specific situation. Every effort has been made to confirm the accuracy of the information presented and to correctly relate generally accepted practices. The authors, editor, and publisher cannot accept responsibility for errors or exclusions or for the outcome of the material presented herein. There is no expressed or implied warranty of this book or information imparted by it. Care has been taken to ensure that drug selection and dosages are in accordance with currently accepted/recommended practice. Due to continuing research, changes in government policy and regulations, and various effects of drug reactions and interactions, it is recommended that the reader carefully review all materials and literature provided for each drug, especially those that are new or not frequently used. Any review or mention of specific companies or products is not intended as an endorsement by the author or publisher.

SLACK Incorporated uses a review process to evaluate submitted material. Prior to publication, educators or clinicians provide important feedback on the content that we publish. We welcome feedback on this work.

Published by: SLACK Incorporated
                  6900 Grove Road
                  Thorofare, NJ 08086 USA
                  Telephone: 856-848-1000
                  Fax: 856-853-5991
                  www.slackbooks.com

Contact SLACK Incorporated for more information about other books in this field or about the availability of our books from distributors outside the United States.

Library of Congress Cataloging-in-Publication Data

101 pearls in refractive, cataract, and corneal surgery / edited by Samir A. Melki and Dimitri T. Azar. -- 2nd ed.
     p. ; cm.
  Includes bibliographical references and index.
  ISBN-13: 978-1-55642-684-1 (alk. paper)
  ISBN-10: 1-55642-684-4 (alk. paper)
  1. Eye--Surgery. I. Melki, Samir A., 1965- II. Azar, Dimitri T. III. Title: One hundred and one pearls in refractive, cataract, and corneal surgery. IV. Title: One hundred one pearls in refractive, cataract, and corneal surgery.
  [DNLM: 1. Ophthalmologic Surgical Procedures. 2. Cataract Extraction. 3. Cornea--surgery. 4. Eye Diseases--surgery. 5. Refractive Errors--surgery. WW 168 Z999 2006]
  RE80.A15 2006
  617.7'1--dc22
                         2006016868

Printed in the United States of America.

Last digit is print number: 10   9   8   7   6   5   4   3   2   1

DEDICATION

To Philip and Alexi who will be able to read and appreciate this dedication in the near future: They will realize that putting together this book would not have been achieved without the support of our friends, family and colleagues, to whom I am most grateful.

S.A.M.

To my teachers and fellows at the Massachusetts Eye and Ear Infirmary;
To my future colleagues, residents, and students at the Illinois Eye and Ear Infirmary;
And to Alexander, Nicholas, Lara, and Nathalie for their overwhelming love and support.

D.T.A.

Contents

ACKNOWLEDGMENTS

We wish to thank the contributing authors of this book, whose hard work has resulted in a more up-to-date text. As in the first edition, we acknowledge the contributions of many unnamed contributors of many pearls discussed in this book. Although we have made every effort to identify the original sources of our pearls, it is likely that several tips and techniques were not adequately referenced; we hope that we will recognize their authors in future editions. The SLACK team has again been tremendously helpful and efficient. We want to particularly thank John Bond, Amy McShane, and Jennifer Briggs for believing in this project from its inception. We are also grateful to Suzanne Miduski for her tireless work in putting the final touches to the second edition.

About the Editors

Samir Melki, MD, PhD: Dr. Melki is the Founder and Director of the Boston Eye Group. He is medical director for ophthalmology at the UK Specialist Hospitals. He is also a clinical instructor at Harvard Medical School and assistant in Ophthalmology at the Massachusetts Eye and Ear Infirmary. Dr Melki completed his ophthalmology residency at Georgetown University Hospital, where he was elected as Chief Resident. This was followed by a fellowship in Corneal and Refractive Surgery at the Massachusetts Eye and Ear Infirmary, where he served as Chief Fellow. His areas of interest include refractive surgery, complex cataract surgery, and ocular surface reconstruction.

Dimitri Azar, MD: Dr. Azar is Professor and Chairman of Ophthalmology at the University of Illinois at Chicago (UIC). After completing his residency, chief residency, and fellowship at the Massachusetts Eye and Ear Infirmary, Dr. Azar became Director of the Refractive Surgery Service at the Wilmer Eye Institute (Johns Hopkins University; 1991-1996). While at the Massachusetts Eye and Ear Infirmary, he was Director of the Corneal and Refractive Surgery Services and Associate Chief of Ophthalmology (1996-2003) and became Professor of Ophthalmology at Harvard Medical School (2003-2006). His research interests include refractive surgery, corneal wound healing, and corneal angiogenesis.

CONTRIBUTING AUTHORS

Natalie A. Afshari, MD
Associate Professor of Ophthalmology
Cornea and Refractive Surgery
Duke University Eye Center
Durham, NC

Esen K. Akpek, MD
Associate Professor of Ophthalmology
Director, Ocular Surface Diseases and Dry Eye Clinic
The Wilmer Eye Institute
Johns Hopkins Hospital
Baltimore, MD

Tushar Agarwal, MD
Assistant Professor
Rajendra Prasad Centre for Ophthalmic Sciences
All India Institute of Medical Sciences
New Delhi, India

Faisal Al-Tobaigy, MD
Research Fellow
Corneal and Refractive Surgery Service
Massachusetts Eye and Ear Infirmary
Harvard Medical School
Boston, MA

Elena Albè, MD
Research Fellow
Corneal and Refractive Surgery Service
Massachusetts Eye and Ear Infirmary
Harvard Medical School
Boston, MA

Rana Altan-Yaycioglu, MD
Assistant Professor in Ophthalmology
Baskent University School of Medicine
Adana, Turkey

Jean-Louis Arné, MD
Professor of Ophthalmology
Director, Cornea and External Diseases, Refractive Services
Hospital Purpan
Toulouse, France

Alexandre Assi, Bsc, MBBS, FRCOphth
Attending Surgeon
Eye and Ear International Hospital
Beirut, Lebanon

Dimitri T. Azar, MD
Professor, Field Chair and Head
Department of Ophthalmology and Visual Science
University of Illinois Eye Center
Chicago, IL

Georges Baikoff, MD
Professor of Ophthalmology
Clinique Monticelli
Marseille, France

Tae-Young Chung, MD
Cornea and Refractive Surgery Service
Department of Ophthalmology
Samsung Medical Center
Sungkyunkwan University School of Medicine
Seoul, South Korea

Elizabeth A. Davis, MD, FACS
Adjunct Assistant Clinical Professor, University of Minnesota
Partner, Minnesota Eye Consultants, PA
Minneapolis, MN

Eric J. Dudenhoefer, MD, Lt. Col., USAF, MC
Assistant Chief, Cornea, External Disease, and Refractive Surgery
Willford Hall Medical Center
Lackland AFB, TX

Michael J. Endl, MD
Fichte-Endl Eye Associates
Director Ophthalmology, Niagara Falls Memorial Hospital
Niagara Falls, NY

C. Stephen Foster, MD, FACS
Founder and President
Massachusetts Eye Research and Surgery Institute
Clinical Professor of Ophthalmology, Harvard Medical School
Boston, MA

Ramon C. Ghanem, MD
Research fellow
Corneal and Refractive Surgery Service
Massachusetts Eye and Ear Infirmary
Harvard Medical School
Boston, MA

Sadeer B. Hannush, MD
Attending Surgeon, Cornea Service
Wills Eye Hospital
Assistant Professor of Ophthalmology
Jefferson Medical College, Thomas Jefferson University
Philadelphia, PA

David R. Hardten, MD
Adjunct Associate Professor, University of Minnesota
Director of Refractive Surgery, Minnesota Eye Consultants
Director of Refractive Surgery, Regions Medical Center
Minneapolis, MN

Thanh Hoang–Xuan, MD
Professor of Ophthalmology
Director, Cornea and External Diseases, Refractive Surgery
Fondation Ophtalmologique A. de Rothschild and Hospital Bichat (AP-HP)
Paris, France

Nada S. Jabbur, MD
Chief of Ophthalmology, Clemenceau Medical Center
affiliated with John Hopkins Medicine International
Beirut, Lebanon

Stephen D. Klyce, PhD
Professor of Ophthalmology and Anatomy
Louisiana State University Eye Center
New Orleans, LA

Richard L. Lindstrom, MD
Clinical Professor, University of Minnesota
Medical Director, Minnesota Eye Consultants
Minneapolis, MN

Richard Mackool, MD
Director, The Mackool Eye Institute
Senior Attending Surgeon, New York Eye and Ear Infirmary
Assistant Clinical Professor, New York Medical College

Pierre G. Mardelli, MD
Glaucoma Service, Department of Ophthalmology
Eye and Ear Hospital, Department of Ophthalmology
Hotel Dieu de France
Beirut, Lebanon

Samir A. Melki, MD, PhD
Director and Founder, Boston Eye Group
Clinical Instructor, Harvard Medical School
Boston, MA

Shahzad Mian, MD
Assistant Professor, WK Kellogg Eye Center
University of Michigan
Ann Arbor, MI

Roberto Pineda II, MD
Director of Refractive Surgery
Cornea and Refractive Surgery Service
Massachusetts Eye and Ear Infirmary
Harvard Medical School
Boston, MA

Jonathan D. Primack, MD
Cornea, External Disease, and Refractive Surgery
Eye Consultants of Pennsylvania
Wyomissing, PA

James J. Reidy, MD, FACS
Associate Professor, Department of Ophthalmology
State University of New York at Buffalo
Buffalo, NY

Ammar N. Safar, MD
Assistant Professor of Ophthalmology
Director, Vitreo-Retinal Service
Jones Eye Institute
University of Arkansas for Medical Sciences
Little Rock, AR

Tohru Sakimoto, MD
Research fellow
Corneal and Refractive Surgery Service
Massachusetts Eye and Ear Infirmary
Harvard Medical School
Boston, MA

H. John Shammas, MD
Clinical Professor of Ophthalmology
University of Southern California, School of Medicine
Los Angeles, CA

Rania M. Shammas, MD
Montefiore Hospital
Albert Einstein University
Bronx, NY

Namrata Sharma, MD
Associate Professor
Rajendra Prasad Centre for Ophthalmic Sciences
All India Institute of Medical Sciences
New Delhi, India

Kimberly C. Sippel, MD
Cornea Consultants of Boston
Boston, MA

Walter J. Stark, MD
Boone Pickens Professor of Ophthalmology
Director, Stark-Mosher Center of Cataract and Corneal Services
The Wilmer Eye Institute
Johns Hopkins Medical School
Baltimore, MD

Rasik B. Vajpayee, MD, FRCSEd
Professor of Ophthalmology
Head Corneal and Cataract Surgery
Centre of Eye Research Australia
University of Melbourne
Melbourne, Australia

Tais Hitomi Wakamatsu, MD
Department of Ophthalmology and Otorhinolaryngology
Faculty of Medical Sciences, State University of Campinas (UNICAMP)
São Paulo, Brazil

FOREWORD

For the first edition of this text, I wrote the following foreword:

"To take on three major topics such as refractive, cataract, and corneal surgery and treat them in a single brief text may seem, at first glance, a bit hazardous, even presumptuous. However, instead of trying to grind through the topics in the traditional way, resulting in superficiality, the authors have cleverly singled out a series of discrete key issues along the cutting edge of this surgery and managed to guide the reader with very sharply focused advice—'pearls.' In this attempt, the authors have clearly succeeded.

"The present volume provides specialists in the various areas an opportunity to digest reports from throughout the world and format the information according to their own considerable experiences. Each chapter focuses on a specific 'how to do it' in a very practical way. The authors are also able to sort out enormous controversies in the field and to superimpose their own good judgment. Considering the enormous worldwide interest in and application of the type of surgery covered, there is no question that this text will be much sought after in the future. In addition, reading it is outright fun!"

For this second edition, which is even more sophisticated than the first, I feel exactly the same way. It should be a natural addition to the library of every anterior segment ophthalmologist who aspires to be at the forefront of our profession.

Claes H. Dohlman, MD
Professor of Ophthalmology
Massachusetts Eye and Ear Infirmary
Harvard Medical School

CHAPTER 1

FOUR
PEARLS FOR SURGICAL PLANNING WITH
CORNEAL TOPOGRAPHY

Stephen D. Klyce, PhD and Michael J. Endl, MD

In the early 1980s, modern corneal topography evolved in response to the need generated by refractive surgery, which was then principally radial keratotomy (RK). Since then, preoperative evaluation with corneal topography has become the standard of care in refractive surgery, and careful screening is essential to successful practice. Subsequently, in the late 1990s, wavefront analysis was added to the surgeon's armamentarium as a means to measure the optics of the whole eye for the more precise laser sculpting of the corneal tissue. While wavefront analysis or aberrometry offers a leap in surgical technology, aberrometers do not replace the more sensitive and broader area coverage of the corneal topographer. Following, we offer a few helpful hints and caveats for the successful use of corneal topography in the optimization of surgical results for the patient and the surgeon.

PEARL #1: KERATOCONUS AND OTHER SUSPECTS

Patients with keratoconus frequently seek out keratorefractive procedures as a means to improve their vision because of the aberrations they often experience with early corneal ectatic changes and the inability of contact lenses and spectacles to provide satisfactory correction. Although less than 0.05% of the general population develops keratoconus, the incidence of keratoconus when refractive surgery is introduced to a region is more than 6% (in some centers, as high as 12%). Patients with mild keratoconus often have asymmetrically-shaped corneas and, for this reason, experience coma with spectacle wear and poor fits with conventional contact lenses. Despite these limitations in refractive correction with appliances, the keratoconus patient should be counseled against seeking a standard surgical refractive alternative. Corneas exhibiting keratoconus signs as well as those with signs of pellucid marginal degeneration have biochemically and structurally altered connective tissue, which renders their corneal stroma susceptible to kerectasia after refractive surgery. While kerectasia may take months or years to develop after tissue removal in refractive surgery, even subtle topographic asymmetry—the earliest sign of keratoconus—should signal caution to the prudent clinician. A normal patient's corneal topography is shown in Figure 1-1; Figure 1-2 illustrates the kerectasia that can result when performing LASIK on a cornea with topographic asymmetry.

With the unfortunate burgeoning in the number of laser in situ keratomileusis (LASIK)-related litigations, it is especially germane to screen patients carefully and to manage topographically suspicious cases appropriately. It is well documented by Randleman and associates that two principle causes of kerectasia after the LASIK procedure for the correction of myopia are too thin a residual stromal bed and preoperative topographic signs of keratoconus. For the higher refractive corrections, surgeons are opting appropriately for the surface ablation techniques of laser epithelial keratomileusis (LASEK) and photorefractive keratectomy (PRK) to circumvent the problem of inadequate residual tissue thickness. When there are questionable signs of keratoconus, some surgeons are also performing LASEK or PRK to avoid the further weakening of the cornea with the creation of the LASIK flap; however, there is at least one report in the literature of kerectasia after PRK. Tissue subtraction refractive procedures, whether under a stromal flap or on the stromal surface, are contraindicated in the presence of signs of corneal ectatic disease. This would include both keratoconus as well as the even less frequent pellucid marginal degeneration.

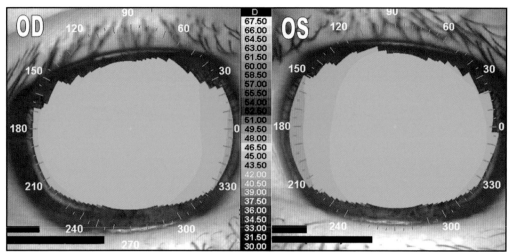

Figure 1-1 (Pearl 1). Corneal topography examination for a topographically normal patient. Note the midline symmetry, uniform central powers, and smooth contours.

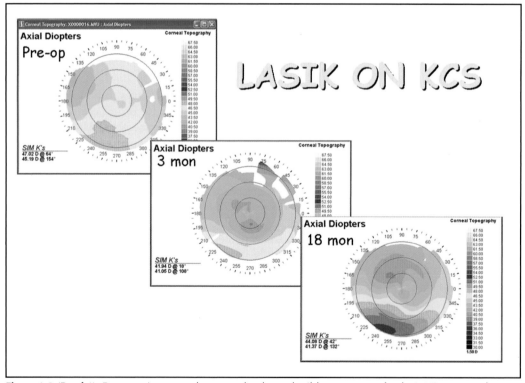

Figure 1-2 (Pearl 1). Preoperative corneal topography showed mild asymmetry of only 1.1 D measured 3 mm below and 3 mm above the corneal apex. Over a period of 18 months, kerectasia ensued, resulting in visual complaints. Eventually, this eye underwent penetrating keratoplasty. Note that the inferior ectasia occurred in the area of the original suspicious steepening. These are displayed with a 1.5 D fixed standard scale. Similar sequelae occur after PRK on keratoconus suspect eyes (R. Zaldivar, personal communication).

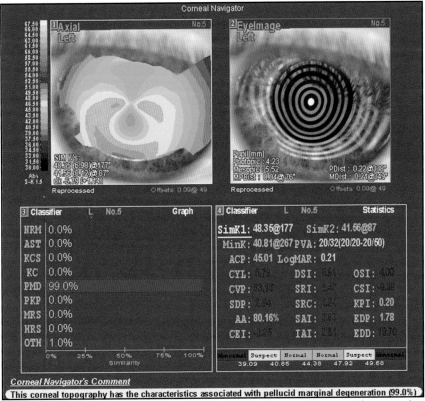

Figure 1-3 (Pearl 1). The NIDEK corneal navigator is able to classify corneal topography, here indicating that the topography is what is normally associated with pellucid marginal degeneration, the hallmarks of which are the vertical negative bow-tie figure and the "C" or claw-shaped region of higher power.

Because of the significant risks to the refractive surgical patient for undetected keratoconus, careful screening with corneal topography plays a critical role in the development and maintenance of a successful refractive surgery practice. Learning to recognize topographic abnormalities is an important first step in this process. Alternatively, new screening software is becoming available using artificial intelligence techniques to assist in preoperative evaluation (Figure 1-3).

The Abnormal Cornea

To this point, we have emphasized the need to screen out the corneal ectatic diseases when considering the candidacy of a patient for the more traditional refractive surgeries. We need to go further and state that any cornea that does not fall within the normal limits of corneal topography should be viewed with caution and the cause of the abnormality ascertained. This raises the question of how to differentiate normal from abnormal topography. With several topography systems, statistical indices are presented along with indications of normal, suspect, and abnormal values (see Figure 1-3). To supplement these utilities, the use of a fixed standard scale with a 1.5-D contour interval is a powerful method used to detect topographic abnormalities because clinically irrelevant detail will be hidden while abnormalities in corneal shape will make themselves known. This point will be amplified further in the following discussion of data presentation.

The Normal Cornea

To detect abnormal topography, it is helpful to recall the features of normal corneal topography: (1) 99.7% (±3 standard deviations) of all normal corneas will have average K-readings within the range

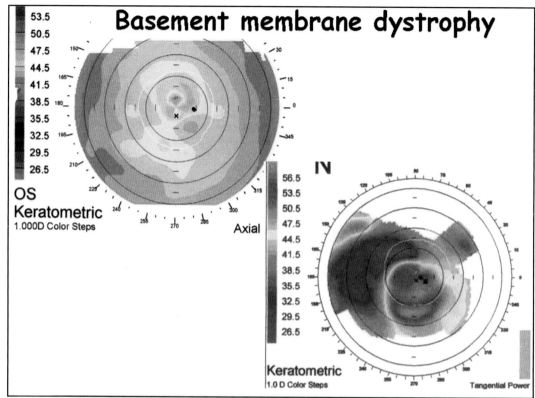

Figure 1-4 (Pearl 1). Preoperative corneal topography (upper left) and several months after LASIK for myopia, this cornea developed a frank kerectasia. The preoperative corneal topography does not have the characteristics of keratoconus or pellucid but is clearly abnormal.

of 39 to 48 D; (2) smooth color map contours occur between power steps with (3) fairly uniform central powers over the photopic pupil and a gradual flattening toward the periphery, particularly in the nasal quadrant; (4) the topography of the two eyes of a patient should be markedly similar, with any features such as corneal astigmatism showing enantiomorphism (mirror image similarity about the midline); and (5) corneal astigmatism, when present, should appear as a symmetric bow-tie with no angulation or skew in the axes between the two lobes of the bow-tie. Characteristics outside these qualities are indicative of abnormal corneal topography. A typical normal patient's exam is shown in Figure 1-1.

Basement Membrane Dystrophy

It is very important in the refractive screening process to understand that keratoconus and its related ecstatic pathologies are not the only concerns. This point can be underscored with a case in which a refractive surgical aspirant underwent screening with unremarkable findings except that irregular contours in corneal topography were present. Perhaps, since the focus of topography screening had been on detecting keratoconus and none of the common signs of an ectatic degenerative disease were found (Figure 1-4), the patient underwent LASIK for myopia. The irregular contours in the corneal power map were due to basement membrane dystrophy. Subsequently, frank kerectasia developed, which will require a corneal transplant in the future. It is becoming clear that corneas with mechanically weak stroma include not only those with keratoconus and pellucid marginal degeneration, but also those with basement membrane dystrophy. Removing tissue from these corneas, whether from under a LASIK flap or from the stromal surface, exacerbates the kerectatic process. Furthermore, since corneal topography is the most sensitive clinical test for the presence of these conditions, a suspicious corneal topography should not be ignored, even when no other clinical signs are present.

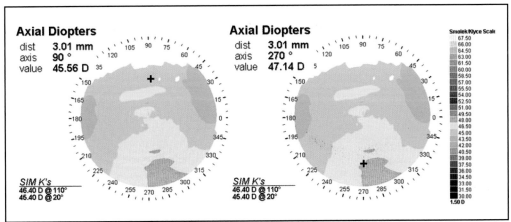

Figure 1-5 (Pearl 1). Using the corneal topographer cursor (black crosses) to estimate the I-S value. For this cornea, the difference between inferior (3 mm at 270 degrees) and superior powers (3 mm at 90 degrees) was 1.58 D. This amount of asymmetry is abnormal. The other eye of this patient, which had even less asymmetry, developed kerectasia after LASIK (see Figure 1-1).

Contact Lenses

One of the confounding variables when evaluating corneal topography is the wearing of contact lenses. It has become customary in some practices to ask patients to discontinue contact lens wear as few as 3 days before screening. In some cases, this may be an adequate period of time, but for those patients who have symptomatic contact lens molding with spectacle blur, studies show that nonwear periods of up to 5 months are necessary for corneas to relax from the molding effects of contact lens wear. In general, patients with a history of contact lens wear and who have abnormal topography should be reevaluated over intervals of 2 to 3 weeks until the corneal topography stabilizes. In any case, these patients should not become candidates for standard refractive surgery unless the topography is stable and normal.

Keratoconus: True or False?

One of the patterns that contact lenses can mold the cornea into is a keratoconus-like pattern with inferior steepening, so it becomes critical to differentiate the true disease from false keratoconus, which has been dubbed pseudokeratoconus. The eyes at greatest risk for pseudokeratoconus are those with corneal astigmatism. In these cases, decentered contact lenses can flatten one half of the topographic bow-tie and allow the other half to steepen. This forms a pattern that can be indistinguishable from true keratoconus. Fortunately, differentiation is fairly straightforward. Discontinue contact lens wear, and a follow-up examination after a 2- to 3-week interval will usually disclose either a symmetrization of the bow-tie for the case of pseudokeratoconus or an actual steepening of the keratoconic figure if the underlying cause is true keratoconus.

Flagging Keratoconus

In the absence of the potentially confounding influence introduced by contact lens wear, several key features of corneal topography can be used for detection. Typically, keratoconus presents as a localized area of inferior steepening. The extent of the steepening consistent with keratoconus is hard to define precisely, yet many use a variant of the Rabinowitz-McDonnell I-S corneal power asymmetry criterion. Although developed to run automatically in conjunction with a corneal topographer, the I-S value can be loosely approximated by subtracting the powers 6 mm apart along the vertical meridian using the moveable cursor normally present with most corneal topographers. A simple rule based on the landmark studies of Rabinowitz and McDonnell is that I-S values greater than 1.4 D but less than 1.9 D would indicate a cornea is suspicious for having keratoconus (forme fruste keratoconus, also called keratoconus suspect [Figure 1-5]). An I-S value 1.9 D or greater would indicate topography consistent with classical

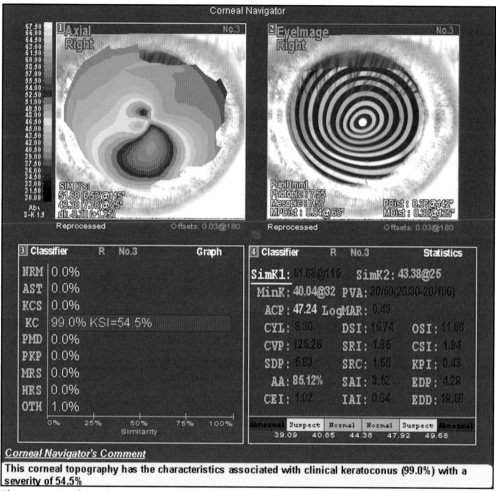

Figure 1-6 (Pearl 1). The NIDEK corneal navigator is able to recognize and classify keratoconus as well as provide an index of severity.

keratoconus. This simple rule is only a guideline. It is important to note that the diagnosis of true keratoconus must eventually rely on the less sensitive but more traditional measures of pachymetry and biomicroscopy. Another common sign of keratoconus includes a more advanced involvement of the disease in one eye compared to the fellow eye and smooth contours in the power map. With contact lens molding effects, the pseudo-keratoconus produced is generally at a similar stage of advancement in both eyes, and there are often associated irregularities in the topographic contours, particularly in the central cornea, consistent with instability of the tear film. While the above-modified I-S detection scheme is extremely useful, more specific automatic tests have been developed for the classification of corneal topography into a number of different categories that include keratoconus (Figure 1-6). These can be powerful screening tools and provide an interactive means to learn corneal topography interpretation.

Variations on a Theme

Keratoconus can present as a variety of patterns on topographic examination. In addition to the more usual pattern of localized inferior steepening, the localized steepening can occur centrally and even entirely within the superior half of the cornea. Keratoconus can also take on the appearance of a steep central, truncated bow-tie, often with skewed axes and giving the appearance of a lazy or drooping figure eight. Finally, keratoconus topography can take the appearance generally presented with pellucid marginal degeneration of a "C" or claw-shaped pattern of elevated power that generally gives rise to against-the-rule astigmatism. In such a case, the arcuate peri-limbal thinning generally associated with pellucid marginal degeneration is absent. Such cases may be most appropriately called topographic pellucid marginal degeneration, with the understanding that the underlying disease is most likely keratoconus.

Always Remember...

The percentage of patients with keratoconus is much higher among refractive surgery candidates than in the general population, but these people and others with pellucid marginal degeneration or basement membrane dystrophy are not good candidates for refractive surgery and must be identified to prevent unsatisfactory results.

The possibility of keratoconus can be indicated with I-S calculations or by using computerized corneal topography classification programs.

If contact lens warpage is suspected, the patient must discontinue lens wear for the period required (up to 5 months may be necessary) for corneal topography to stabilize in order to optimize preoperative data for refractive surgery.

PEARL #2: ORBSCAN FOR A POSTERIOR PERSPECTIVE

Unlike the traditional corneal topographer that measures only corneal front surface shape, the B&L Orbscan (Bausch & Lomb, Rochester, NY) scanning slit elevation topographer is designed to provide elevation data from both the anterior and posterior corneal surfaces. The current model, Orbscan IIz, incorporates a Placido disc as well to provide traditional high-resolution corneal front surface power maps. The combination approach permits estimates of corneal thickness across the corneal surface, which can be useful for both preoperative and postoperative evaluations. The standard four-map display can include wide area corneal pachymetry along with anterior and posterior enhanced elevation maps and standard corneal topography (Figure 1-7). When attempting to interpret the elevation images, it is important to remember that the Orbscan's elevation data are derived from height differences of best-fitting spheres. Thus, the elevation maps are referred to as "float" maps and look different from (in fact, almost the opposite of) conventional axial curvature maps. In the cornea analyzed in Figure 1-7, an inferior localized area of lower surface power appears as an elevation on the anterior float map. This difference in presentation format may be difficult to use in clinical evaluations and could draw attention away from critical details. For example, in the examination shown in Figure 1-7, note the unusual area of inferior low power in the axial map and the thinner-than-expected inferior pachymetry. This cornea is an example of topographic pellucid marginal degeneration, and following LASIK for myopia, this patient experienced visually debilitating kerectasia.

The repeatability of the Orbscan's pachymetry has been shown to be comparable to that of manual ultrasound measurements. It should be noted, however, that the Orbscan thickness measurements can vary (by approximately 5%) from those of ultrasound pachymetry. There is no agreed-upon conversion factor to date, and Orbscan pachymetry values should not be directly substituted with ultrasound measurements. An additional caveat is that each unit can be set to use a different standard calibration factor, so readings can vary from one screening site to another.

With the LASIK procedure, it is thought that ectasia of the cornea may occur if the depth of the resection (cap thickness plus the maximum thickness of tissue removed during ablation) is more than 50% of the corneal pachymetry. The Orbscan's LASIK Safety Nomogram software is designed to calculate residual bed thickness during the planning stage and may recommend a smaller microkeratome plate size or caution against the procedure if too great a depth is calculated. One advantage this instrument could have over manual central point pachymetry is in patients where the thinnest regions of the

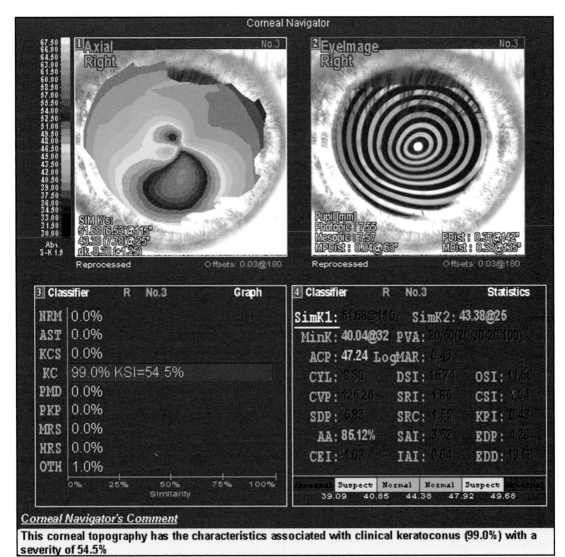

Figure 1-7 (Pearl 2). Standard Orbscan topography and pachymetry display. Data for A and B are obtained with scanning light slits. (1) Anterior float is a display of the difference between the front corneal surface elevation and a reference sphere. (2) Posterior float is a display of the difference between the posterior corneal surface elevation and a reference sphere. (3) Axial corneal topography measured with the Placido feature. (4) Two-dimensional thickness profile based on the slit scans. Note the unusual inferior depression in C, the posterior inferior protrusion in B, and the relatively thin inferior pachymetry shown in D. After LASIK, this cornea experienced kerectasia. Interpretation: topographic pellucid marginal degeneration.

cornea may be off center. Here, the central ultrasound measurements may be misleading, resulting in a thinner residual stromal bed thickness than anticipated. However, the surgeon must also bear in mind the consistent bias in pachymetry values produced by the Orbscan. Thus, for corneas on the thin side of normal, we recommend that the surgeon err on the side of caution and use conventional ultrasound data for residual bed thickness estimates. At the same time, we also recommend that corneas with ultrasound central thickness below 490 μm (microns) be excluded from refractive surgery altogether.

Always Remember...

Because the Orbscan's relative elevation measures height differences from a best-fitting sphere, the appearance of the resulting maps is opposite that of the conventional axial curvature maps (ie, steeper regions are displayed as minus and flatter regions as plus elevations).

The Orbscan's pachymetry measurements have an adjustable bias, which may make the data not directly comparable to ultrasound pachymetry values. There is no agreed-upon conversion factor, so Orbscan pachymetry values cannot be used interchangeably with ultrasound measurements.

PEARL #3: SO MANY MAPS, SO LITTLE TIME

In corneal topography, the axial power map is the traditional presentation format used clinically, particularly for diagnostics. This is provided by all current corneal topographers and was chosen because measurement in terms of diopters (D) of power is familiar from traditional keratometry. Also, the axial power map as will be seen below represents corneal curvature in the same manner that clinicians think of corneal power—uniformly steep centrally with flattening toward the periphery. Although there is ongoing controversy as to which presentation format is most useful for the clinician, the axial power map, using a carefully developed and tested scale, is essential and it should be the base presentation format learned because other displays can mask pathology, as will be shown.

Besides the axial power maps, there are three other common ways to present corneal topographic information:

1) Refractive corneal power maps (Figure 1-8) use ray tracing to account for spherical aberration. This calculation provides a more accurate presentation of corneal power but is misleading in terms of true corneal curvature or shape. Additionally, it presents a format containing more contour intervals for normal corneas instead of the uncomplicated appearance one obtains with the axial power map. The major danger in using this format is that peripheral corneal topographic pathology (including keratoconus and pellucid marginal degeneration) can be masked (Figure 1-9), allowing inappropriate refractive correction measures to be taken.

2) Instantaneous radius of curvature power maps (also called tangential or meridianal maps) present the local corneal curvature as calculated from mathematical derivatives of the corneal surface that result in a very noisy map (Figure 1-8). As a result, the data are not clinically useful for preoperative screening. However, this very sensitive scheme is particularly useful for optimizing the transition zone in the development of laser refractive surgery algorithms, as the transition zone is emphasized producing the so-called "red ring."

3) Corneal elevation maps can be obtained directly with fluorescein profilometry or with the scanning slit technology (Orbscan). Elevation maps can also be obtained from Placido disk topographers (Figure 1-8). Direct display of elevation data is not useful, as the distortions in the corneal surface are too subtle to provide diagnostic information. Presentation of total wavefront error has the same limitation, since the low-order terms of refractive error (defocus) and cylinder usually dominate the map. However, elevation data can be enhanced through the subtraction of a reference sphere, as is done with the Orbscan "float" maps, to magnify details such as the depth of an ablation following myopic excimer laser surgery. It is important to understand that whether elevation maps are created with the Orbscan or calculated from Placido data, their appearance will be altered by the shape of the reference surface that is subtracted. Most often, this shape (usually a sphere) is not the same even between repeated exams of the same eye and cannot be chosen by the user. This limits its clinical utility.

Most corneal topographers come with an array of map styles and layouts. Among these are single maps, multiple maps, and special purpose maps, such as the difference map, which is a very useful corneal topography utility. The difference map (Figure 1-10) is most often used to subtract two power maps, presenting this difference along with the originals. The difference map can be extremely useful in evaluating

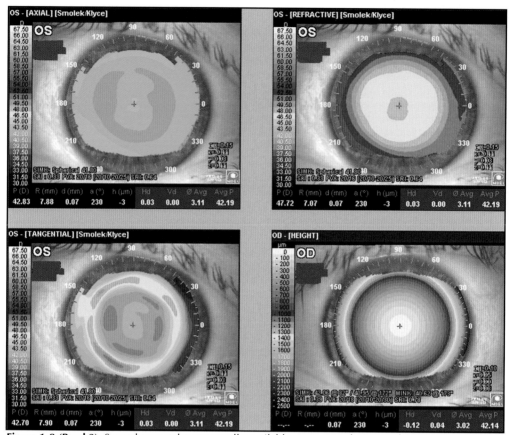

Figure 1-8 (Pearl 3). Several map styles are usually available on a corneal topographer. Here, a LASIK for myopia with prolate treatment zone is analyzed with the four most common topography displays. The beginning user of corneal topography should start by using the axial power map with a fixed, standard scale (upper left). The refractive power map is shown in the upper right, the instantaneous power map in the lower left (note the "red ring"), and an elevation map is shown in the lower right.

the effect of a refractive procedure on the shape of the cornea. For refractive surgery patients, difference maps can be used to establish preoperative topographic (and refractive) stability. In particular, contact lens wearers can undergo molding that produces 1 D or more of refractive shift, which can take up to 6 months to resolve. A comparison of difference maps over this time period can establish the patient's readiness for treatment.

The appearance of central islands following excimer laser ablations for myopia can be accurately measured postoperatively with the power difference map by subtracting a postoperative exam from the preoperative cornea. Central islands, which can occur with both PRK and LASIK, generally resolve with time, and the time course of these changes can be accurately analyzed with difference maps. One can also use the difference map to evaluate unwanted stromal remodeling after refractive surgery. When shopping for a topographer, one should always be concerned about the repeatability of the measurements. This can easily be ascertained using the topographers' difference map. Noting that fixation nystagmus is unavoidable and will always result in a slight rotational difference between sequential exams, one should be looking for less than 0.25-D difference over most of the corneal difference map as an index of repeatability.

In summary, the number of different styles of topography maps can be bewildering. A surgeon needs to become familiar first with the fundamentals of corneal topography before attempting to use this information in keratorefractive procedures. Furthermore, because the many available machines have yet to

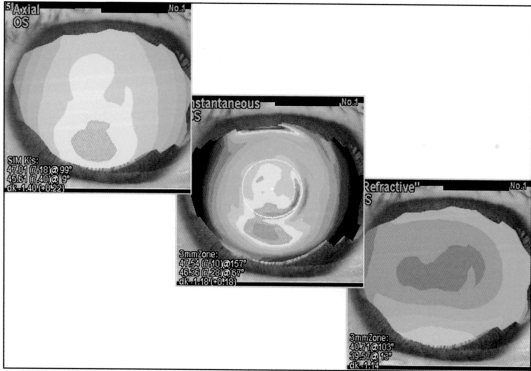

Figure 1-9 (Pearl 3). The axial power map (upper left) is most useful for clinical interpretation of corneal topography. In the case of mild keratoconus, the instantaneous power map (center) offers only confusing noise to the map, while the refractive power map (lower right) actually hides the inferior ectasia, causing the clinician to miss the interpretation of keratoconus.

adopt a universal standard, the physician should become comfortable with one machine and one map format for optimal clinical use. We recommend the axial map coupled with a fixed, standard scale such as the one proposed by Smolek and Klyce as the starting point with any topographer.

Always Remember...

The number of topography maps can be bewildering. There is no universal standard yet; the physician should become familiar with one machine and one map format for optimal clinical use.

The difference map subtracts two power maps and presents this difference along with the originals. Use difference maps to establish preoperative stability and postoperative results.

PEARL #4: CAREFUL ALIGNMENT IS NOT OPTIONAL IN REFRACTIVE SURGERY

To correct cylindrical errors, precise alignment of the refractive procedure with the patient's astigmatic axis is challenging but extremely important. Cyclotorsion of the eye occurs with different gaze positions, with upright versus supine positions of the body, and with anxiety. Whether one is considering photorefractive astigmatic keratectomy (PARK), LASIK, LASEK, or astigmatic keratectomy (AK), an accurate location of the eye's steep meridian is the first step in the process, but marking this axis directly on the eye or relating its position to iris features with computer image analysis will greatly improve predictability.

Initially, it must be determined whether the subjectively measured astigmatism matches the objective measurements. The magnitude and axis of the topographic astigmatism and keratometry readings are

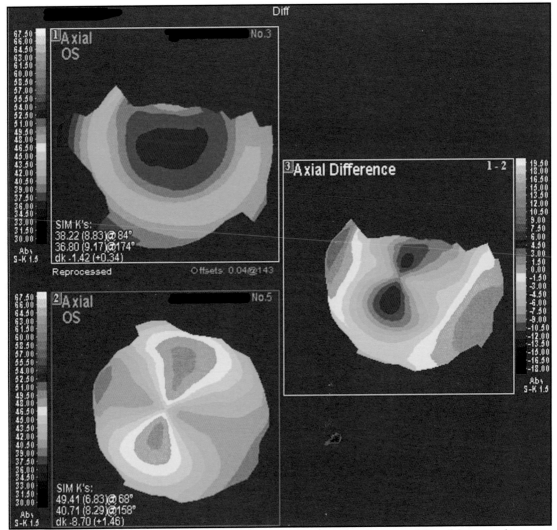

Figure 1-10 (Pearl 3). The axial difference map can be useful for examining the repeatability of the corneal topographer and changes in topography with time. Here, the postoperative result (upper right) shows excellent quality after an astigmatic LASIK correction on an eye with nearly 9 D of corneal cylinder. The change in curvature is shown in the right-most panel.

most often equal to that of the refractive astigmatism at the corneal plane since the cornea is usually the source of most of the ocular aberrations. If there is a significant difference, the values should be rechecked. Remaining differences may be due to lenticular astigmatism or posterior corneal anomalies, and the refractive astigmatism should be used to set the surgical magnitude and axis.

With the increasing popularity and success of wavefront guided laser ablations, preoperative axis alignment and registration are more important than ever. After all, "garbage in = garbage out." Preoperative axis markings in eyes undergoing PARK have demonstrated better postoperative outcomes than their unmarked counterparts. This is especially true if the astigmatic treatment is 1.25 D or greater. As we attempt to include astigmatism with the treatment of higher order aberrations, the tolerance for the eye's misalignment decreases. Previous studies with corneal topography and direct measurement have shown an average of about 4 degrees and a maximum of about 15 degrees of positional cyclorotation.

The impact of axis misalignment on the magnitude of astigmatic correction is shown in Figure 1-11. A 10-degree error in cylinder axis alignment will result in a 30% reduction in cylindrical correction.

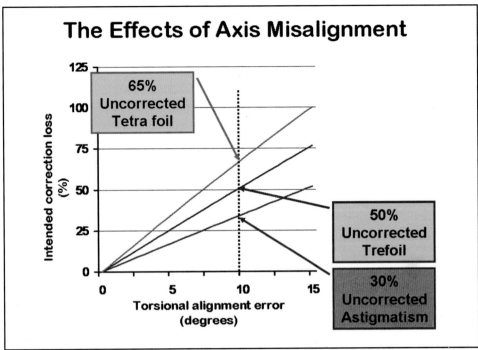

Figure 1-11 (Pearl 4). Effects of rotational axis misalignment on correction of cylinder, trefoil, and tetrafoil. Not compensating for cyclotorsional movements during refractive surgery can negate many, even all of the intended corrections. (Courtesy of Alcon Laboratories, Inc.)

Concerning wavefront-guided ablations, the error is substantially larger for the higher-order aberrations. For example, for trefoil, a 10-degree misalignment would produce a 50% reduction in correction while for tetrafoil, the error rises to 65%. At even higher orders, cyclotorsional errors can virtually eliminate the benefit of wavefront correction.

In refractive surgery, torsional errors are generally attributable to two factors. The most important is the degree of cyclorotation or cyclotorsion when a patient lies down. This averages about 4 to 5 degrees, with cyclotorsion in some patients reaching 10 degrees or more. The second factor is intraoperative cyclotorsion. This is typically about 1 or 2 degrees at most and usually has a negligible effect. Clearly, accounting for cyclotorsion in the eye is important to obtain a good conventional result and even more critical when wavefront-guided correction is attempted. The different laser systems implement alignment and registration systems for both conventional astigmatic surgery and for wavefront-guided correction. These often use fiducial reference lines and marks and iris landmarks to remove the measurement-to-surgery cylcotorsion effects. The alignment of the eye to the laser is perhaps the most important step for the surgeon to obtain good results with astigmatic corrections and particularly with higher-order corrections.

To ensure optimum alignment during surgery, it is helpful to use a surgical marker at the slit lamp. By marking the limbus at the 6 and 12 o'clock positions while the patient is in the same erect viewpoint as with the phoropter, possible torsional shifts elicited when changing to a supine position can be avoided. These marks can then be aligned with most laser reticules through gentle manipulation of the patient's head. It is not usually necessary to mark the steep axis specifically because this information will be incorporated in the ablation profile, but doing so will provide a further means to verify accuracy of the induced cylinder axis.

To this point, we have addressed only rotational alignment in refractive surgery. In reality, alignment has 5 dimensions: X, Y, Z, rotation, and time. The time dimension relates to the adequacy of the laser tracking system to maintain the laser reference position relative to the position of the eye during the course of the ablation procedure. The Z position relates to maintaining the optimum distance between the laser head and the corneal surface. In most configurations, the excimer laser beam is only slightly divergent along the Z-axis, making this dimension less critical. The x and y dimensions relate to centration of the refractive surgical procedure.

Optical zone decentration has been linked to postoperative complaints involving glare, halos, and decreased best-corrected visual acuity (BCVA). Previous investigations have shown a high subjective tolerance to decentration in myopic ablations (at least for daytime vision), probably because of the fairly uniform power distribution in the treatment zone. However, hyperopic and astigmatic corrections require a higher degree of accuracy because decentrations of only 0.5 mm may be symptomatic postoperatively. Thus, reliable centration in these patients is essential. Furthermore, mesopic conditions can exacerbate the visual symptoms of decentration for all refractive surgeries.

Careful technique and topographic evaluation can be used to optimize centration. Before and during surgery, several steps can be taken to ensure appropriate alignment of the optical zone. Because pupil does not dilate and constrict symmetrically (miosis tends to shift the center nasally), Uozato and Guyton teach us that the laser ablation should be centered over the natural entrance pupil of the eye. In patients with a large angle lambda, many surgeons center the refractive procedure on a point midway between the center of the entrance pupil and the corneal reflex. With good technique, many beginning surgeons are able to achieve centrations averaging 0.4 mm, although with experience, this can be improved to a mean of 0.2 mm. As with rotational errors, centration errors will reduce the effectiveness of treating the higher-order aberrations.

Patient anxiety, which leads to loss of fixation, can be greatly reduced through careful preoperative preparation. This involves a thorough explanation of the treatment, including a videotaped or live viewing of the procedure so the patient may become familiar with the positioning and sounds of the microkeratome/laser. Medications such as benzodiazepines and adjustments to the surgical chair may further aid patient comfort and encourage fixation.

During the procedure, the surgeon should ensure that the patient's face is square to the laser by means of gentle support and manipulation of the head. The patient is encouraged to maintain fixation on a flashing light target. To avoid confusion, the surgeon should dim the microscope light and make certain that the patient has definitively identified the target light prior to initiation of the procedure. The surgeon then uses the laser's optical centration device for centering. This varies from laser to laser (eg, a red alignment reticule is used in the VISX lasers). For larger corrections, significant drying or welling of fluid may occur on the ablation surface, interfering with both the surgeon's view of the pupil and the patient's ability to fixate. Placing preoperative limbal markings with gentian violet at the x and y coordinates (a four-cut RK marker works well) supplements the surgeon's orientation with the laser reticule. In addition, stopping the procedure and temporarily replacing the LASIK flap may be necessary to realign patient fixation.

Finally, as noted above, several of the lasers incorporate sophisticated eye tracking systems that promise to reduce the aberrations that can be induced by eye movements during the course of the surgery. However, the desired center must be established by the surgeon, and care must be taken throughout the procedure that the tracking is continuing. Even with the tracker operational, it is important to take steps to minimize eye movement. This is because trackers generally key on the pupil margin or the iris features, and since these elements are in a different plane than the cornea, rotation will cause the cornea to move greater distances than the tracking plane.

How well a refractive surgical treatment was centered over the pupil can be assessed with corneal topography. Generally, when examining a color map, the pupil is outlined by the software. On some units, the coordinates of the entrance pupil and the diameter are provided automatically. On others, a measuring cursor is available that one can use to determine the pupil center. This is done by positioning the cursor successively at the pupil margin along the 0, 90, 180, and 270 degree semi-meridians and recording the distances in millimeters. The x and y coordinates for the pupil center will then be calculated from one-half the sum of the readings at 0 and 180 degrees and one-half the sum of the readings at 90 and 270 degrees, respectively. Next, the center of the treated area is determined. This is generally done by displaying the corneal topography with the most sensitive contour interval available (0.5 D or less, for example). Then, a template (made of a series of concentric circles centered on x and y axes drawn on transparent overhead projection material) is held against the computer monitor so that one of the circles most closely approximates the circular borders of the treated area. With the borders aligned with the template, the screen cursor is positioned underneath the origin of the x and y axes, and a reading of this center is found. Finally, the amount of treatment decentration is calculated from the distance between the center of the pupil and the center of the treated area using a straightforward trigonometric relationship.

Perhaps the development of a real-time corneal topography system that allows the refractive surgeon to objectively assess alignment during the procedure will help eliminate decentration errors in the future.

Always Remember...

If the subjectively measured astigmatism is not equal to the objective measurements, the remaining differences may be due to lenticular astigmatism or posterior corneal anomalies, and the refractive astigmatism should be used in the surgical plan.

For incisional AK, conventional K readings tend to underestimate the amount of cylinder to be corrected. Rely on corneal topography for increased accuracy, and remember to treat the steep meridian (or the axis of the 'plus' cylinder).

By marking the limbus at the 6 and 12 o'clock positions while the patient is in the same erect viewpoint as with the phoropter, possible torsional shifts elicited when changing to a supine position can be reduced.

The pupil does not dilate and constrict symmetrically (miosis tends to shift the center nasally). Therefore, we suggest using the natural pupil for refractive procedures.

Decentration can be evaluated with corneal topography.

Studies have shown that careful planning and surgical experience can reduce average decentration by half.

Patients with myopic corrections are tolerant of decentration in the daytime. Caveat: patients with hyperopic and astigmatic corrections and/or mesopic conditions are less tolerant to decentration that can result in complaints of poor vision.

BIBLIOGRAPHY

Almendral D, Waller SG, Talamo JH. Assessment of ablation zone centration after photorefractive keratectomy using a vector center of mass formula. *J Refract Surg.* 1996;12:483-491.

Alpins NA. Vector analysis of astigmatism changes by flattening, steepening, and torque. *J Cataract Refract Surg.* 1997;23:1503-1514.

Auffarth GU, Wang L, Volcker HE. Keratoconus evaluation using the Orbscan Topography System. *J Cataract Refract Surg.* 2000;26:222-228.

Consultation section. Refractive surgical problem. *J Cataract Refract Surg.* 1998;24:876-881.

Farah S, Olafsson E, et al. Outcome of corneal and laser astimatic axis alignment in photoastigmatic refractive keratectomy. *J Cataract Refract Surg.* 2000; 26:1722-1728.

Liu Z, Huang AJ, Pflugfelder SC. Evaluation of corneal thickness and topography in normal eyes using the Orbscan corneal topography system. *Br J Ophthalmol.* 1999;83:774-778.

Rabinowitz YS, McDonnell PJ. Computer-assisted corneal topography in keratoconus. *Refract Corneal Surg.* 1989;5:400-408.

Randleman JB, Russell B, Ward MA, Thompson KP, Stulting RD. Risk factors and prognosis for corneal ectasia after LASIK. *Ophthalmology.* 2003;110:267-275.

Schwartz BH, Hersh PS. Corneal topography of Phase III excimer laser photorefractive keratectomy. *Ophthalmology.* 1995;102:951-962.

Smith EM, Talamo JH. Cyclotorsion in the seated and supine patient. *J Cataract Refract Surg.* 1995;21:402-403.

Smolek MK, Klyce SD. The Tomey/computed anatomy TMS-1 videokeratoscope. In: Gills JP, Sanders DR, Thornton SP, Martin RG, Gayton JL, Holladay JT, eds. *Corneal Topography: The State of the Art.* Thorofare, NJ: SLACK Incorporated; 1995:123-149.

Smolek MK, Klyce SD. Current keratoconus detection methods compared with a neural network approach. *Invest Ophthalmol Vis Sci.* 1997;38:2290-2299.

Smolek MK, Klyce SD, Hovis JK. The universal standard scale: proposed improvements to the ANSI standard corneal topography map. *Ophthalmology.* 2002;109:361-369.

Smolek MK, Oshika T, Klyce SD, et al. Topographic assessment of irregular astigmatism after photorefractive keratectomy. *J Cataract Refract Surg.* 1998;24:1079-1086.

Srivannaboon S, Reinstein DZ, Sutton HF, et al. Accuracy of Orbscan total optical power maps in detecting refractive change after myopic laser in situ keratomileusis. *J Cataract Refract Surg.* 1999;25:1596-1599.

Suzuki A, Maeda N, Watanabe H, et al. Using a reference point and videokeratography for intraoperative identification of astigmatism axis. *J Cataract Refract Surg.* 1997;23:1491-1495.

Uozato H, Guyton DL. Centering corneal surgical procedures. *Am J Ophthalmol.* 1987;103:264-275.

Vajpayee RB, McCarty CA, Taylor HR. Evaluation of the axis alignment system for correction of myopic astigmatism with the excimer laser. *J Cataract Refract Surg.* 1998;24:911-916.

Wilson SE, Lin DT, Klyce SD, Reidy JJ, Insler MS. Topographic changes in contact lens-induced corneal warpage. *Ophthalmology.* 1990;97:734-744.

Wilson SE, Klyce SD. Screening for corneal topographic abnormalities prior to refractive surgery. *Ophthalmology.* 1994;101:147-152.

Wilson SE, Klyce SD, Husseini ZM. Standardized color-coded maps for corneal topography. *Ophthalmology.* 1993;100:1723-1727.

Wilson SE, Klyce SD, McDonald MB, et al. Changes in corneal topography after excimer laser photorefractive keratectomy for myopia. *Ophthalmology.* 1991;98:1338-1347.

Yayli V, Kaufman SC, Thompson HW. Corneal thickness measurements with the Orbscan Topographay System and ultrasonic pachymetry. *J Cataract Refract Surg.* 1997;23:1345-1350.

Zadok D, Haviv D, Vishnevskia-Dai V, et al. Excimer laser photoastigmatic refractive keratectomy: eighteen-month follow-up. *Ophthalmology.* 1998;105:620-623.

CHAPTER 2

FOUR
PEARLS IN WAVEFRONT TECHNOLOGY

Tohru Sakimoto, MD and Dimitri T. Azar, MD

Until recently, the purpose of conventional refractive surgery has been to correct defocus and astigmatism. Unsatisfied patients, complaining of halos, reduced low contrast visual acuity (especially in dark situations), and/or restricted visual performance, often experienced postoperative increase in high-order optical aberrations. These include coma, spherical aberrations, and secondary astigmatism, which can be detected by wavefront testing and can be minimized by custom refractive surgery.

PEARL #5: WAVEFRONT TECHNOLOGY AND ABERROMETRY

In physical optics, light is considered as a wave that spreads in all directions; a wavefront is like a ripple that is in phase when a stone is thrown into water. A wavefront describes light rays emanating from a source and represents an isochronous surface shape (ie, all the points along the rays that are in phase). It measures the optical path in its entirety and is not limited to any given refractive surface. Thus, the wavefront describes the aggregate effects of the optical system of the eye causing distortions in the wavefront from the image. In the absence of wavefront aberrations, the wavefront would exit the eye as a perfect plane that is perpendicular to the visual axis. On the other hand, when optical aberrations are present, as is true in all eyes, the wavefront would form a surface rather than a plane. Wavefront aberrations are defined as the deviation between the wavefront surface originating from a given optical system and the hypothetical wavefront plane originating from an ideal optical system (Figures 2-1 to 2-8). For a given eye, the shape of the wavefront is a fundamental and unique description of the optical quality of the whole eye.

Wavefront analysis assesses the optical quality of the eye by evaluating the shape of its wavefront and provides detailed maps of the eye's optical quality at every point in the pupil. It expresses the deformity of wavefront shape in three-dimensional space (see Figure 2-1). The unit used in wavefront analysis is micrometers or fractions of wavelengths and is often displayed as the root mean square. Alternatively, the influence of aberration on retinal image quality can be simulated by computing the point-spread function using Fourier transforms (see Figures 2-2 to 2-8).

Wavefront aberrations are usually expressed mathematically in polynomial expansions. Zernike developed a set of polynomial equations and applied them for the analysis of wavefront properties of optical systems. Zernike decomposition breaks the wave aberration into its component aberrations. A multitude of optical aberrations exists, and they are usually grouped into two major categories: lower-order and higher-order aberrations. There are three components to the lower-order aberrations: zero order (a constant), first order (tilt or prism), and second order (defocus and astigmatism). Lower-order aberrations can be corrected with glasses, contact lenses, and conventional refractive surgery. Higher-order aberrations are simply fit to a more complex wavefront shape. They represent smaller irregularities in the optical system of the eyes, representing about 17% of the total optical error in humans. Some of the more common higher-order aberrations include third order (coma and trefoil), fourth order (spherical aberration and secondary astigmatism), fifth order (including secondary coma), and sixth order (including secondary spherical aberration). Polynomials can be expanded up to any arbitrary order if sufficient numbers of measurements for calculations are made. Using the Zernike coefficients of each

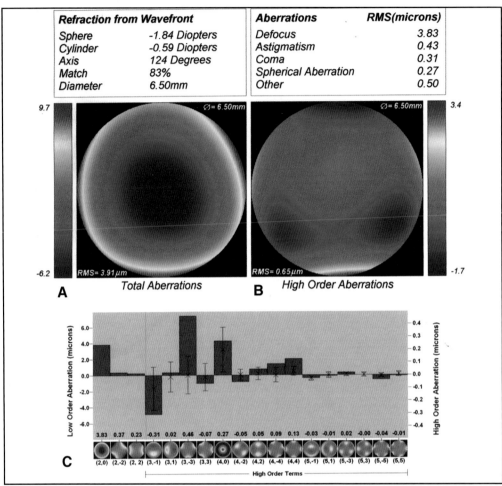

Figure 2-1 (Pearl 5). Hartmann-Shack aberrometry in a patient with low myopic astigmatism (Alcon) showing (A) total aberrations and (B) with low myopic astigmatism. (C) The aberrations could be resolved to the various Zernike terms of differing magnitudes. In C, the first three terms represent the second- (lower) order aberrations and are displayed on a -6 μm to +6 μm scale. The other terms (third order and beyond) are displayed using a scale of -0.4 μm to +0.4 μm.

term, monochromatic aberrations can be evaluated quantitatively. The understanding of the clinical significance of many of the higher-order aberrations is still in its infancy. Spherical aberration and coma can result in reduced quality of vision, but the effects of other higher aberrations are less understood.

Always Remember...

   Zernike decomposition of the ocular wavefront identifies the magnitude of various lower- and higher-order aberrations of the eye.

PEARL #6: DIAGNOSTIC VALUE OF ABERROMETRY

   Wavefront analysis may be used to evaluate postoperative visual disability after refractive surgery. The increase of higher-order aberrations after conventional refractive surgery may be responsible for the reduction of contrast sensitivity (CS) and reduced quality of vision.

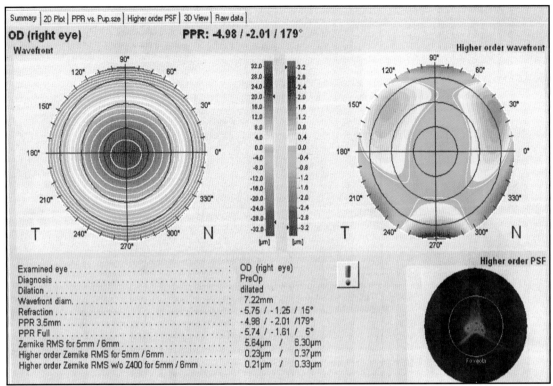

Figure 2-2 (Pearl 5). Aberrometry of the right eye of a patient with moderately high myopic astigmatism (Zywave) showing (A) the total aberration and (B) the higher-order aberrations (C) with their corresponding point spread function (PFS).

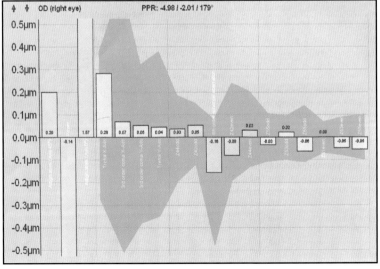

Figure 2-3 (Pearl 5). Graphic representation of the magnitudes of the second-order Zernike polynomials (first three bars) and the higher-order polynomials of the eye in Figure 2-2.

Figure 2-4 (Pearl 5). Recalculation of the sphere (blue) and cylinder magnitude (red) and axis (yellow) for the eye in Figure 2-2. Note the trend for increasing myopia with increased pupil diameter.

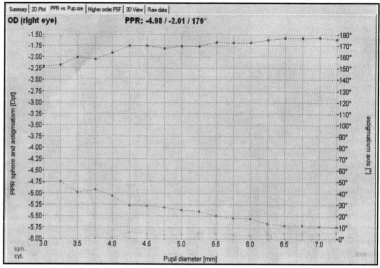

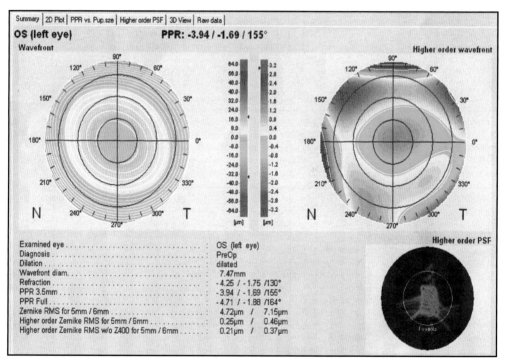

Figure 2-5 (Pearl 5). The contralateral left eye of the patient in Figure 2-2 showing (A) total and (B) higher-order aberrations. (C) The PSF of the higher order aberrations is more diffuse than that in Figure 2-2.

Wavefront analysis provides various maps that represent specific information regarding aberrations expressed in microns of deviation from plane wavefront. This analysis shows not only lower-order aberrations that are typified by myopia, hyperopia, and astigmatism but also higher-order aberrations such as coma, secondary astigmatism, etc. Lower-order aberrations can be corrected with spectacles, contact lenses, intraocular lenses (IOLs), and various refractive surgeries by successfully correcting the sphere and cylinder. Other optical phenomena, such as the unavoidable effects of pupil-dependent diffraction, may limit sharpness of the retinal image.

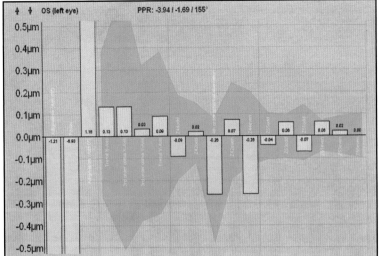

Figure 2-6 (Pearl 5). The Zernike polynomial display corresponding to Figure 2-5 and showing -0.26 µm of spherical aberrations (and quadrafoil).

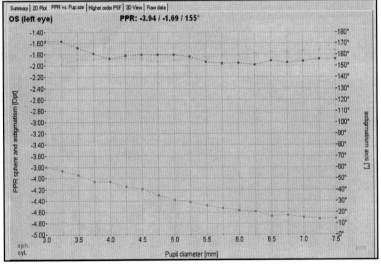

Figure 2-7 (Pearl 5). Recalculation of the myopia and astigmatism of the eye shown in Figure 2-5, showing ~1 D myopic shift with increasing pupil diameter from 3 to 7.5 mm.

Despite differences in their operating principles, wavefront analyzers usually use ray-tracing methods to trace the path of multiple light rays through the individual eye to reconstruct the wavefront. In general, the wavefront sensors can be classified into three types: (1) in-going retinal imaging aberrometry, as in Tscherning and sequential retinal ray tracing method; (2) out-going wavefront aberrometry, as is used in the Hartmann-Shack aberrometer; and (3) in-going feedback aberrometry, as in skiascopy and the spatially resolved refractometer.

The commercial aberrometers in use today are based on the three main methods of wavefront sensing: outgoing reflection (Hartmann-Shack), ray imaging (ray tracing/Tscherning), and ingoing adjustable refractometry (spatially resolved refractometer). The Hartmann-Shack sensor, which the three principal United States Food and Drug Administration (FDA)-approved wavefront-guided laser platforms (Technolas 217z Zyoptix System by Bausch & Lomb [Rochester, NY], LADARVision system by Alcon [Fort Worth, Tex], and Wavescan by VISX [Santa Ana, Calif]) are based on, projects a laser light utilizing approximately 200 spots into the eye to illuminate a small spot on the retina. The probe light reflected from the fovea is imaged onto the Hartmann-Shack sensor, which consists of a matrix of small lenslets. These lenslets sample corresponding areas of the pupils and divide the wavefront into

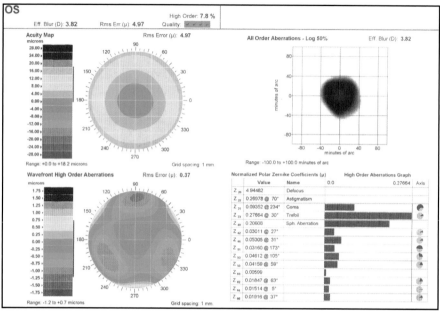

Figure 2-8 (Pearl 5). Custom Vue (VISX, Santa Clara, Calif) aberrometry showing (A, B) the total aberrations and (C) the higher-order aberrations. (D) Graphic representations of the higher-order aberrations suggest that trefoil (Z33) and spherical aberration (Z40) are the highest.

individual beams, producing multiple images of the same retinal spot of light to form a spot pattern that is focused onto a CCD camera. The deviation of each spot from its corresponding lenslet axis is used to calculate the aberrations.

Always Remember…

In contrast to corneal topography, which measures the aberrations created by the corneal surface, wavefront sensing measures the total refractive error including aberrations of the entire optical system of the eye, including those resulting from the anterior surface of the cornea, as well as additional aberrations emanating from the posterior corneal, lens, and retina.

PEARL #7: ADVANTAGES OF CUSTOMIZED REFRACTIVE PROCEDURE

Wavefront-guided LASIK and LASEK may have several advantages over conventional LASIK techniques (Figure 2-9). One of the benefits is the potential to reduce postoperative night vision problems. Wavefront-guided LASIK and LASEK may decrease the amount of induced aberrations and prevent preexisting aberrations, especially among higher-order aberrations. Also, the use of a small spot scanning laser with eye tracking in wavefront-guided ablations may result in the possibility of the so-called supervision in which postoperative UCVA may exceed the preoperative BCVA.

The main goal of a customized refractive procedure is to correct all aberrations of the eye and, therefore, to improve the visual acuity, especially under scotopic conditions. Thus, one obvious advantage of correcting the optical aberrations in the eye is the potential for creating an optically perfect image.

Optical customization relies on accurate measurement of an optical aberration profile and its transfer to a reliable laser aberration system for the customized ablation with high fidelity (see Figures 2-8 and 2-9). There are two approaches to optical customization in refractive surgery: corneal topography-guided and wavefront-guided ablation. Anatomic considerations include individual structural variations of the eye that are relevant to refractive surgery, such as corneal diameter and thickness and pupil size under

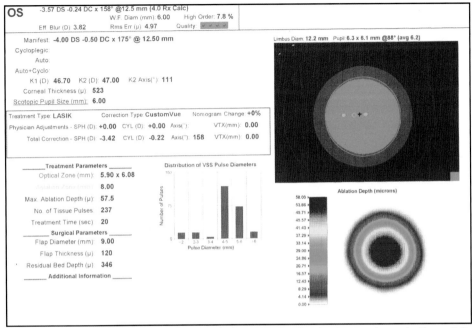

Figure 2-9 (Pearl 7). Custom (wavefront-guided) LASIK planning for the eye shown in Figure 2-8. The treatment parameters are enumerated (left) and are displayed with regards to the pupil position (upper right) and ablation profile (lower right).

different lighting conditions. In general, these factors may influence the visual outcome to a lesser degree than the optical parameters. Nonetheless, anatomic factors such as anterior chamber depth, axial length, and the lens shape may be incorporated into customized ablations in the future. Functional consideration may influence the acceptance of customized corneal outcomes in a given patient and thus should be considered in the surgical strategy. These include patient occupational and recreational needs, age, refraction, and psychophysiologic tolerance.

Always Remember...

Wavefront analysis does not provide all the necessary information for corneal ablation. Comparison with the manifest and/or cycloplegic clinical refraction is important to minimize unpredictable refractive outcomes.

Pearl #8: Limitations of Wavefront-Guided LASIK and LASEK

The major limitation of wavefront-guided LASIK ablations is that this technology cannot predictably compensate for surgically induced higher-order aberrations following primary custom LASIK. One alternative is to perform customized LASEK surgery, in which the surgically induced higher-order aberrations are less, especially when the epithelial thickness after LASEK approximates the preoperative thickness.

The variability of visual outcomes after wavefront-guided LASIK may result from the differential corneal wound healing, flap effect, and biomechanical response. These factors contribute to the surgically induced higher-order aberrations after customized LASIK surgery. Other important practical difficulties include inherent technical difficulties and limitations in accurately measuring ocular aberrations in a given eye, compensation for cyclotorsion during laser treatment, and precise centration. Moreover, the location of the pupil center can change under photopic, mesopic, and pharmacologically dilated conditions. Wavefront aberrations occur because of local deviation in the path of light entering the eye through different points in the pupil. With larger pupils, the higher-order aberrations are greater. Although the changes in centration are typically slight, significant changes have been observed. In these instances, there could be large changes in the refractive state of the eye as the curvature of the cornea changes with location. Moreover, optical aberrations differ for various wavelengths of light. Current wavefront aberration quantification is based on monochromatic systems. In our natural, polychromatic world, the optical quality and visual performance may be better predicted by polychromatic system. However, chromatic aberrations cannot be corrected with current refractive surgical techniques because these errors are inherent to the properties of the optics rather than its shape.

Always Remember …

Wavefront aberrations contribute to the decrease in visual acuity in patients with large pupils, especially at night. Although the correction of such aberrations should theoretically improve mesopic vision performance, the current limitations of wavefront-guided LASIK and LASEK interfere with our ability to achieve these results consistently.

BIBLIOGRAPHY

Chalita MR, Finkenthal J, Xu M, Krueger RR. LADARWave wavefront measurement in normal eyes. *J Refract Surg.* 2004;20:132-138.

Cheng X, Thibos LN, Bradley A. Estimating visual quality from wavefront aberration measurements. *J Refract Surg.* 2003;19: S579-S584.

Cosar CB, Saltuk G, Sener AB. Wavefront-guided laser in situ keratomileusis with the Bausch & Lomb Zyoptix system. *J Refract Surg.* 2004;20:35-39.

Sakimoto T, Rosenblatt M, Azar DT. Laser eye surgery for refractive errors. *Lancet.* 2006;367(9520):1432-1447.

Yamane N, Miyata K, Samejima T, et al. Ocular higher-order aberrations and contrast sensitivity after conventional laser in situ keratomileusis. *Invest Ophthalmol Vis Sci.* 2004;45:3986-3990.

Yeh PC, Azar DT. Wavefront-guided custom LASIK and LASEK: techniques and outcomes. In: Foster CS, Azar DT, Dohlman CH, eds. *Smolin and Thoft's The Cornea: Scientific Foundations and Clinical Practice.* Philadelphia, PA: Lippincott Williams & Wilkins; 2004:1257-1268.

CHAPTER 3

SEVEN
PEARLS IN LASIK TECHNIQUES WITH MK
AND INTRALASE

Elizabeth A. Davis, MD, FACS; David R. Hardten, MD; and Richard L. Lindstrom, MD

This chapter describes surgical techniques designed to achieve the best outcomes and lowest risk of complications in LASIK surgery using the microkeratome and the Intralase Femtosecond laser. A rigorous, methodical, and skilled approach is the key to success in refractive surgery. LASIK surgery is a quick, highly regimented procedure. However, this does not imply that it is rote or without thought. Each case is unique, and the surgeon must be prepared at all times to handle challenging situations.

PEARL #9: PREOPERATIVE COUNSELING AND INFORMED CONSENT

A successful LASIK surgery depends as much on a technically good operation as it does on an appropriately counseled patient. Patients do not like visual surprises. If they are forewarned about potential postoperative visual disturbances, these will be less disconcerting to them.

It is important to set realistic expectations. It is far better to counsel for lesser outcomes and have the patient pleasantly surprised than the converse. The goal of the surgery is functional vision without glasses or contact lenses. Thus, one should counsel for 20/40 vision and not 20/20 vision. The vast majority of the time, outcomes will be better than this, and the patient will be pleased.

For patients in the presbyopic age group, a discussion of the need for reading glasses should occur. For surgeons who aim for some initial overcorrection, the patient should also be forewarned about some difficulty with their intermediate range of vision. Myopic patients need to understand that their faces might be blurry in the mirror postoperatively. Hyperopic patients should be informed that they might be temporarily myopic.

The surgeon should explain that visual recovery, particularly for the higher levels of correction, might take from several weeks to months. Although a big improvement in their uncorrected visual acuity (UCVA) will occur in the first 24 hours, continued improvement can occur after this. Additionally, patients should understand that 5% to 10% will require an enhancement to achieve the desired results. They should be given an estimate of the time at which this might occur.

Always Remember...

It is far better to counsel for lesser outcomes and have the patient pleasantly surprised than the converse.

PEARL #10: ACHIEVE ADEQUATE EXPOSURE AND ACHIEVE AND CONFIRM ADEQUATE SUCTION

Achieving adequate exposure is critical to visibility, achieving adequate suction, ability to place the microkeratome properly, unobstructed passage of the microkeratome, and a well-exposed stromal bed. There are certain types of orbital anatomy that may predispose to difficulty with exposure. For example, deep set orbits, prominent brows, or small palpebral fissures may interfere with placement of instruments on the globe. These findings should all be noted preoperatively. In these instances, as well as others, it is often helpful to have the patient maintain a chin-up position for adequate visibility and instrument placement. If the patient has a prominent lower cheek that overhangs the lower blade of the speculum,

Figure 3-1 (Pearl 10). Adequate exposure is essential to allow unimpeded microkeratome movement. The lashes may be covered with a surgical drape. A Chayet drain (Becton Dickinson, Franklin Lakes, NJ) can be used around the limbus to prevent migration of debris into the stromal interface.

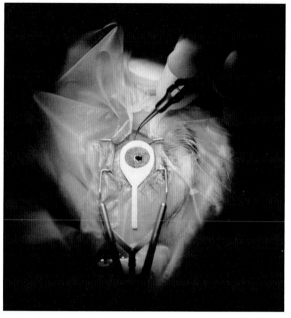

the surgeon may use his or her fourth and fifth fingers to retract this tissue inferiorly and out of the surgical field. Similarly, a technician can assist with this maneuver.

The lashes should be isolated from the surgical field. Not only is this important for sterility purposes, but it prevents cilia from being caught in the keratome. Simply placing tape or steristrips over the lashes achieves this isolation of lashes. A Tegaderm (3M Corp, St. Paul, Minn) adhesive plastic also works well. If cut in half, one half can be used for the upper lid and the other half for the lower lid. Another option is to use a surgical drape (Figure 3-1), or one may simply use a closed-bladed speculum.

Placement of the suction ring may be facilitated by gently pressing down on the speculum. This causes the globe to proptose and results in greater exposure. Additionally, once adequate suction has been achieved, one can carefully lift the eye up and out of the orbit with the suction ring to allow unobstructed passage of the microkeratome.

In cases of small palpebral fissures, it is often useful to have several lid specula available. Often, switching from a closed-bladed speculum to an open-bladed one may provide the few millimeters needed to insert the suction ring.

Exposure is sometimes limited primarily by eyelid squeezing. The vast majority of these situations are easily circumvented by proper instruction to the patient and a calm, reassuring demeanor. Also, specula with a screw or locking mechanism counteract squeezing much better than self-retaining specula. Nevertheless, in a few cases, it may not be possible to get the patient to relax the eyelids. In such a situation, one might consider a facial nerve block. Less frequently, and only with the patient's consent, one might perform a lateral canthotomy. Rarely, some surgeons have reported doing a retrobulbar injection in order to proptose the globe.

Achieving and confirming adequate suction is necessary in creating a proper flap. Loss of suction or inadequate suction can result in a short flap, a small flap, a free cap, a buttonhole, or an irregular edge. As mentioned above, good exposure is critical. If it is not possible to seat the suction ring on the globe unobstructed, vacuum cannot be obtained. Additionally, a prolonged struggle to fit the instruments onto the eye can lead to conjunctival chemosis and either inability to obtain suction or pseudosuction. Pseudosuction is when the vacuum registers high because the conjunctiva or drapes are occluding the suction holes. In this case, the intraocular pressure (IOP) will not be sufficiently elevated to pass the microkeratome.

It is important to seat the suction ring properly on the globe, then apply firm, even pressure. Once this is done, suction can be applied.

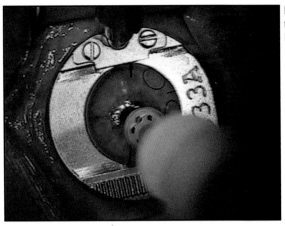

Figure 3-2 (Pearl 10). Measurement of IOP after suction activation with a pneumotonometer. (Courtesy of Dimitri T. Azar, MD.)

There are several indicators of sufficient suction. No single indicator should be relied upon alone. Rather, the surgeon should observe for several of them. First, the sound of the pump changes when adequate suction is achieved. Secondly, the vacuum pressure should register as greater than 25 mm Hg (millimeters of mercury). Additionally, the pupil will dilate slightly. If asked, the patient will report that his or her vision has dimmed or blacked out. The surgeon may use tonometry to confirm that the IOP has risen. Commonly used devices include the Barraquer tonometer (Ocular Instruments, Bellevue, Wash) or a pneumotonometer (Figure 3-2). Lastly, one can confirm good suction if the globe can be elevated out of the orbit by lifting up gently on the suction ring. This should be done prior to IOP measurement to avoid inadvertent loss of suction.

After adequate suction has been achieved and confirmed, it is important to not torque or pull on the suction ring to any great extent. Such maneuvers can result in immediate loss of suction. Some surgeons like to reconfirm suction after the microkeratome has been engaged.

Always Remember...

After adequate suction has been achieved and confirmed, it is important to not torque or pull on the suction ring to any great extent.

Gentle pressure on the lid speculum may help proptose the globe to achieve adequate exposure in patients with small palpebral fissures.

PEARL #11: CREATE A COMPLETE FLAP AND USE INTRALASE WHEN APPROPRIATE

The incidence of flap complications should be less than 0.1% with the newer microkeratomes in experienced hands, especially with the Intralase Femtosecond laser. Some flap complications are the result of unusual corneal anatomy. For example, corneas steeper than 46.00 D may buckle during the keratome pass, leading to buttonholed or centrally thinned flaps. This complication can be essentially eliminated with the Intralase Femtosecond laser. Corneas flatter than 41.00 D are more prone to free caps with mechanical microkeratomes. Keratometry readings should be noted preoperatively and used to select the appropriate ring size. A smaller, deeper mechanically generated flap should be made when corneas are unusually steep, and a larger flap should be created for flat corneas. These limitations are not needed for Intralase-generated flaps.

It is understood that careful inspection of the microkeratome (blade, gears, flap receptacle) is crucial to avoiding flap complications. In the case of the Intralase, the cone head should be applied over the cornea and centration should be attempted, avoiding the limbal vascular arcade. The equipment should be meticulously cleaned and assembled.

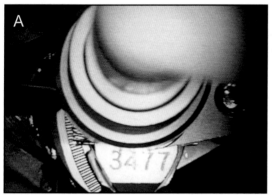
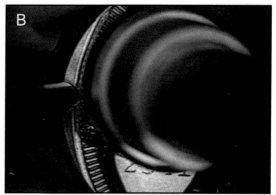

Figure 3-3 (Pearl 11). The Hansatome gear stops at a two-teeth distance from the end of the underlying smooth track, indicating complete dissection of the corneal flap when using an 8.5-mm suction ring. The gear travels the two-teeth distance, and the underlying smooth track cannot be seen when using a 9.5-mm suction ring.

As mentioned previously, adequate exposure is necessary to allow unimpeded passage of the microkeratome. Both the surgeon and assistant should check that the lids, lashes, and drapes are clear of the surgical field prior to the forward pass of the keratome. In keratomes where the flap cannot be visualized as it is dissected, certain visual clues may help ensure a complete pass. When an 8.5-mm Hansatome ring (Bausch & Lomb Corporate, Claremont, Calif) is used, a two-teeth gap can be seen on the gear track above the underlying smooth platform, indicating that the pass is complete (Figure 3-3). In contrast, no gap is seen with the 9.5-mm ring.

If resistance is met during the forward passage of the keratome or the keratome comes to a stop, the surgeon should stop and examine the field. Are the drapes caught in the speculum? Is the patient squeezing, or is the speculum in the way? Any obstruction should be gently removed, and care should be taken to not torque the suction ring off the eye. If no obvious obstruction is found, then the surgeon can tap, tap, tap on the forward foot pedal of the microkeratome. Sometimes, this allows the motor to overcome some temporary resistance. If this is not possible, then the microkeratome should be reversed and removed from the eye even if an incomplete pass has been made. One should never reverse the microkeratome and go forward. This can result in the blade penetrating to a deeper level than the initial pass. A case of anterior segment perforation has occurred when the surgeon reversed the microkeratome part way and then proceeded forward again.

With the Intralase, attention should be focused on flap centration, adequate meniscus size, and clearing of the meniscus by the laser beam. This would ensure adequate flap creation. If an opaque bubble layer (OBL) is noted, the flap is lifted 15 to 20 minutes later. This avoids interference with the eye-tracking device of the excimer laser.

Always Remember...

Achieve adequate centration with the Intralase and delay flap lifting if OBL occurs.

Never back up and go forward again with the microkeratome (it is OK to tap, tap, tap forward).

PEARL #12: ACHIEVE CONSISTENT HYDRATION

To achieve an appropriate ablation depth, the hydration of the stromal bed needs to be adjusted in the same manner for all cases. Too much moisture results in overhydration, less tissue removed per pulse of the laser, undercorrection, or irregular astigmatism. Too little moisture results in an excessively dry bed, more tissue ablation per pulse of laser, and overcorrection. After the flap has been created and prior to turning it back, the top of the cap should be wiped. This prevents any excess fluid from getting onto the stromal bed as the flap is lifted. Some surgeons prefer forceps to lift the flap rather than a cannula, which can drip fluid.

Some surgeons prefer to treat with the bed moist, while others like it drier. Which method one chooses is not important, but it is critical to be consistent and develop a nomogram based on that particular technique. In very humid or dry climates, it may be necessary to intermittently pause during the ablation to adjust the hydration of the stroma if there is excessive moisture or drying as the ablation proceeds. Using the ring light and high magnification will best allow the surgeon to determine the hydration status. It is much more difficult to follow fluid patterns without the ring light.

Excess pooling of fluid can often be found on the stromal bed near the hinge after folding back the flap, and this should be wicked away with a soft surgical sponge. Likewise, any bleeding from the vessels of a peripheral pannus should be wiped away. If a soft surgical sponge is touched near the edge of the area of bleeding during the treatment, it may be possible to wick away the blood periodically without having to stop the laser. A smaller flap size may also be used to avoid cutting through these vessels. Some surgeons have reported success in using a drop of phenylephrine, apraclonidine, or brimonidine just prior to the procedure to constrict these vessels. However, this should be done with caution. If too much time passes, pupil dilation can occur with phenylephrine. Additionally, some cases of slipped flaps have been reported when apraclonidine or brimonidine was used. A useful alternative is naphazoline 0.012% (eg, Naphcon-A [Alcon Laboratories, Fort Worth, Tex]), which allows vascular constriction with a slower mydriatic action.

In all situations, the surgeon should try to minimize the amount of time between turning the flap and ablating. Focus and centration should be adjusted and treatment numbers checked prior to lifting back the flap. Once the flap is lifted, the stromal hydration is adjusted, and patient fixation is achieved, the ablation should proceed.

Always Remember…

In contrast to phenylephrine, naphazoline minimizes bleeding from limbal vessels while avoiding pupillary dilation.

PEARL #13: PERFORM THE APPROPRIATE ABLATION

Performing the correct ablation is the surgeon's responsibility. The original clinical work-up with refraction and topography should be brought to the operating room. The cylinder orientation should be checked against the topography. If the axes are vastly different, particularly if the power of the cylinder is significant, this should be double checked with a second refraction (preferably prior to bringing the patient into the laser suite).

If it is necessary to transpose the cylinder format before entering the refraction into the laser or in order to perform a nomogram adjustment, then special care must be made to ensure that the axis is shifted appropriately.

Multiple checks by both the surgeon and technician can reduce the incidence of errors. The surgeon and technician should check the numbers prior to entering the laser suite and again after the nomogram adjustment has been performed. One final check can then be performed by having the technician hold the chart next to the laser screen. Both the technician and surgeon should then check that the numbers entered into the laser are correct. This is done for the first eye before gloving and for the second eye before the flap is created. It is also helpful to read aloud the patient's name and eye to be treated. This way, no errors are made by using the wrong chart or switching the treatments for the eyes.

Always Remember…

Performing the correct laser ablation is the surgeon's responsibility.

Pearl #14: Reposition the Flap

Debris can originate from multiple sources. Meibomian oil and makeup from the lids, lint from surgical sponges, particles from the microkeratome, and debris from the cannula or irrigating fluid can all accumulate beneath the flap. In order to prevent these particles from gaining access to the surgical field, certain measures can be taken. First, the surgeon should examine the lids preoperatively and treat ocular surface disease aggressively. Warm soaks, a topical antibiotic, or even systemic doxycycline should be considered to treat meibomian gland disease. Patients should be instructed to carefully remove makeup prior to surgery and clean the lids and lashes the night before and morning of the surgery.

Some surgeons consider irrigating the ocular surface prior to surgery, but this can sometimes stir up more meibomian particles. However, this may be useful to wash away other debris. Some surgeons like to place a Chayet sponge (Becton Dickinson, Franklin Lakes, NJ) around the cornea after the flap is created to isolate the stromal bed from the rest of the surgical field (see Figure 3-1). The ring is moistened with a balanced salt solution and applied around the limbus after the fornices are dried with a Weck cell and following the removal of the suction ring. In eyes with small palpebral fissures, the flat end of the ring is trimmed to ease placement and avoid lifting by the lid in superior-hinged flaps. If this is done, it is important to carefully monitor hydration to ensure no pooling of fluid is induced with the presence of a sponge.

Once the ablation is performed and the flap replaced, a cannula should be used to irrigate beneath the flap. The cannula should be moved back and forth beneath the flap to loosen any particles that adhered to the stromal bed or back of the flap. Excess irrigation should be collected with suction, a suction speculum, a microsponge, or a drain. Overly aggressive irrigation should be avoided, however, to prevent cap edema and retraction of the flap edges.

The surgeon should carefully inspect the flap interface using high magnification and side illumination to ensure all debris has been removed. Some surgeons prefer to examine the patient once more at the slit lamp prior to discharging the patient. If any significant debris is noted, the flap can be relifted and irrigated.

Always Remember...

Lint fibers may float in the atmosphere and settle at the stromal interface. This can be minimized by the use of scrub suits by the surgical team and moistening gauze material in the surgical field.

Proper flap alignment is crucial to preventing striae. Striae are problematic when they are prominent and centrally located. In these cases, striae can result in irregular astigmatism and poor UCVA as well as a loss of best-spectacle-corrected acuity.

Marking the cornea prior to creating the flap can help in aligning the flap after the ablation. However, excessive marking should be avoided to prevent epithelial toxicity. Also, the surgeon should be aware that if the epithelium shifts during passage of the microkeratome, the marks might not line up. A more important indicator of proper flap alignment is gutter symmetry. Once the flap is turned over, care should be taken to make sure it is neatly positioned in the fornix or on the lid speculum. It should not be folded over on itself or wrinkled. If this occurs, a significant crease can develop across the flap, which may be difficult to smooth out.

Various instruments are available to iron the flap, but simply stroking or painting the flap back into position with a moistened surgical sponge can achieve an excellent result. Initially stroking the flap from the hinge toward the opposite direction does this. Once good alignment is achieved and the flap begins to adhere, gentle stroking may be performed in oblique directions in a radial fashion. Surgeons that are more aggressive may use a drier sponge to perform stretching by placing the sponge on the flap edge and pulling in a radial direction. The ring light is very useful in identifying striae. One can see discontinuities in the reflection rather than a smooth continuous circle of light (Figure 3-4A). Refloating the flap will allow it to settle into correct position (Figure 3-4B). As mentioned above, excessive

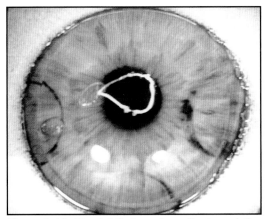

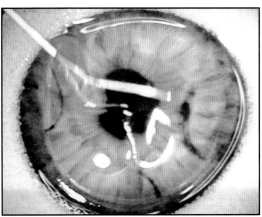

Figure 3-4A (Pearl 14). Irregular reflection of the microscope light and unmatched fiducial marks are strong indicators of a misaligned LASIK flap.

Figure 3-4B (Pearl 14). Refloating the flap with balanced salt solution on a cannula will allow adequate repositioning.

irrigation should be avoided because this can lead to cap swelling, retraction from the edges of the bed, and gutter asymmetry. These flaps can be difficult to align and are more prone to striae postoperatively.

The surgeon should also ensure that the flap adheres well to the underlying stromal bed before removing the lid speculum. There are several options available for drying the cornea. The flap may be allowed to simply air dry. This should be done for 3 to 5 minutes. Alternatively, with some lasers (such as the VISX laser [VISX Incorporated, Santa Clara, Calif]), the surgeon may turn on the vacuum for 30 to 60 seconds to dehydrate the flap. Filtered low-power compressed air or oxygen may be directed onto the epithelium for 10 to 20 seconds. Over-drying should be avoided because this can result in cap retraction and striae.

Good adhesion can be confirmed with the striae test. Using a dry Merocel sponge (Medtronic Solan, Jacksonville, Fla) or other blunt instrument, gentle pressure is applied downward on the epithelium just beyond the keratectomy. If good adhesion is present, fine folds will radiate into the flap.

Lubrication should be applied to the cornea prior to removing the lid speculum. This will reduce friction from the lid postoperatively as the patient blinks and decreases the risk of flap displacement.

Care should be taken not to displace the flap in removing the speculum. As the speculum is closed, it should be lifted upward off the globe. The patient should be instructed not to squeeze on speculum removal. Once the speculum is out, the surgeon should have the patient open his or her eyes once more to inspect the flap position.

Always Remember...

If the epithelium shifts during the microkeratome passage, the fiducial dye marks may not be as reliable for adequate flap positioning.

Good flap adhesion can be confirmed with the striae test. This may in itself cause flap striae and should be used cautiously.

PEARL #15: AVOID AND TREAT LOOSE EPITHELIUM

Loose epithelium may be encountered intraoperatively after the microkeratome makes its pass. Most commonly, this is found near the flap hinge, but occasionally, it can involve a more diffuse area of the flap surface. Patients may be predisposed to this complication if they have evidence of anterior

Figure 3-5 (Pearl 15). Epithelial defect in a LASIK flap noted after the keratome pass. (Courtesy of Nada S. Jabbur, Wilmer Eye Institute.)

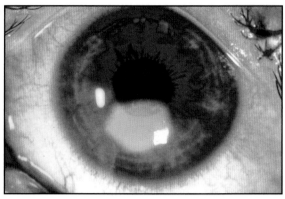

basement membrane dystrophy and/or recurrent erosions. A careful history depicting any prior episodes of spontaneous eye pain should be sought. A thorough slit lamp examination should be performed to look for epithelial abnormalities. In severe cases, topography will show irregular astigmatism.

It is crucial to avoid epithelial toxicity. The surgeon should limit the use of preoperative anesthetic drops. No more than two drops per eye should be applied. Additionally, marking of the cornea should be done sparingly because the ink is toxic to the epithelium. A lubricating drop should be placed on the corneal surface just prior to the microkeratome pass.

One method that appears to decrease the incidence of epithelial defects with the Hansatome microkeratome is to release suction on the reverse pass. This allows the flap to unroll under no tension. Gentle downward pressure with the suction ring prevents the patient from moving his or her eye during these few seconds.

If loose epithelium is encountered after the flap is repositioned appropriately, it should be manipulated back into place with a microsponge. If this is not possible or if loose epithelium is an impediment to stroking the flap, it should be removed with forceps or a dry microsponge. For central or large epithelial defects (Figure 3-5), a bandage contact should be placed. This is typically left in position for a week until the surface is completely re-epithelialized.

Always Remember…

There is a higher incidence of diffuse lamellar keratitis (DLK) with LASIK flap epithelial defects. Consider using stronger and/or more frequent postoperative topical steroids to prevent DLK.

BIBLIOGRAPHY

Carlson KH, Carpel EF. Epithelial folds following slippage of LASIK flap. *Ophthalmic Surg Lasers.* 2000;31(5):435-437.

Davis EA, Hardten DR, Lindstrom RL. LASIK complications. *Int Ophthalmol Clin.* 2000;40(3):67-75.

Holland SP, Srivannaboon S, Reinstein DZ. Avoiding serious corneal complications of laser assisted in situ keratomileusis and photorefractive keratectomy. *Ophthalmology.* 2000;107(4):640-652.

Shah MN, Misra M, Wihelmus KR, Koch DD. Diffuse lamellar keratitis associated with epithelial defects after laser in situ keratomileusis. *J Cataract Refract Surg.* 2000;26(9):1312-1318.

Tham VM, Maloney RK. Microkeratome complications of laser in situ keratomileusis. *Ophthalmology.* 2000;107(5):920-924.

Updegraff SA, Kritzinger MS. Laser in situ keratomileusis technique. *Curr Opin Ophthalmol.* 2000;11(4):267-272.

von Kulajta P, Stark WJ, O'Brien TP. Management of flap striae. *Int Ophthalmol Clin.* 2000;40(3):87-92.

CHAPTER 4

Six Pearls
in Prevention and Management of
LASIK Complications

Samir A. Melki, MD, PhD and Dimitri T. Azar, MD

This chapter describes several techniques to prevent and manage complications of LASIK. We will review ways to address unexpected problems encountered either during or after the procedure. Potentially serious complications can be successfully addressed if ways to manage them are thought through ahead of time.

PEARL #16: THE MIDCUT JAM, THE SLIDING SUCTION RING, AND THE FREE CAP

The suction ring has fit well, the keratome slides easily in place, and the cut is proceeding smoothly until… it stops halfway and does not respond to either forward or backward pedal commands (Figure 4-1). This unpleasant situation occurs secondary to a mechanical or electrical failure of the keratome. The main goal of the surgeon in this situation is to protect the flap and the stromal bed from the keratome blade. Resuming forward movement may result in an uneven cut; however, if the blade has passed beyond the treatment margin, resuming forward movement would not compromise visual acuity.

A quick check of electrical wiring may reveal a loose connection, especially at the connection with the keratome motor. For the Hansatome, if no movement can be initiated, carefully releasing suction and sliding the keratome-suction ring as one unit backward will ensure that the flap is not incarcerated under the blade. The keratome head cannot be reversed along the track manually. Every keratome should be handled differently in this situation, and the surgeon should inquire about the best approach to handle such a situation.

Application of adequate suction is essential for dissection of good quality corneal flaps. On occasion, the suction ring slides prior to the buildup of adequate vacuum, and the flap is decentered relative to the pupillary axis. Applying equal downward pressure on the ring through its handle and at the base knob for 3 to 5 seconds prior to initiating vacuum may minimize this problem.

The initial vacuum may still result in a decentered ring with a large slant, requiring the surgeon to release the vacuum and reposition the ring. It is not uncommon to see the ring sliding back in the conjunctival groove created by the initial suction. Intentional decentration of the ring in the opposite direction prior to activating suction may achieve better centration because the vacuum level may be high enough by the time the ring slides close to the center to prevent further slide toward the initial groove.

Another approach is to change the ring size (eg, from 8.5 to 9.5 mm), hence avoiding the chemotic conjunctiva. Some surgeons advocate applying Vasocon-A (Alcon Laboratories, Fort Worth, Tex), allowing a decrease in conjunctival swelling, and reattempting the procedure 30 minutes later. If this does not resolve the conjunctival chemosis, further difficulties might be encountered, and it is best to delay the surgery for another day.

A free cap results from unintended complete dissection of the corneal flap by the microkeratome head. In certain instances, the microkeratome can jam, preventing head reversal. This might prompt the surgeon to release the suction, thus, lifting the instrument with an incarcerated flap, resulting in a free cap. Intraoperative factors leading to a free cap are the same as those leading to a thin or perforated flap, namely poor blade-to-cornea coupling. This is especially true for flatter corneas, which are more

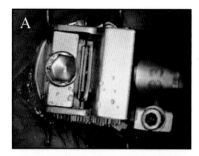

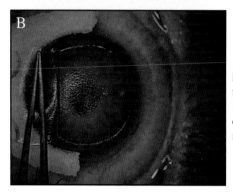

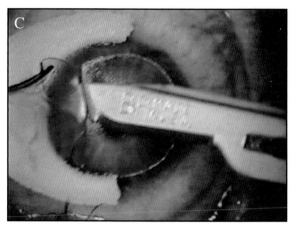

Figure 4-1 (Pearl 16). Incomplete flap: (A) The keratome forward travel is obstructed by the lid speculum, (B) resulting in an incomplete flap. (C) Attempting to manually extend the flap with a blade is a risky maneuver and may result in flap perforation.

prone to smaller cap formation. Other maneuvers, such as malpositioning and/or misadjusting of the flap thickness footplate during assembly of certain microkeratomes, can lead to a free cap.

If the cap is trapped in the keratome head, it should be gently retrieved, stretched, and kept well hydrated. If the diameter of the exposed stroma is adequate, laser ablation may proceed as usual. When recovered, a cap can be repositioned using the preplaced marks to allow proper orientation and can be allowed additional time to adhere compared to a hinged flap. A bandage contact lens is helpful to tamponade the cap and to prevent slippage upon lid contact. Patching the eye may prevent loss of the contact lens and the underlying flap. Suturing is rarely necessary.

A small cap (ie, smaller than the optical zone) should prompt the surgeon to replace it in position and avoid the laser ablation. If the cap cannot be recovered, the epithelium will grow centrally as after other "superficial" keratectomy procedures and may result in a significant hyperopic shift and possible irregular astigmatism. Laser treatment is deferred until refractive stability is achieved.

Always Remember...

Tape the eyelid closed overnight to prevent the loss of a free cap, even with the concurrent use of a contact lens. Patching the eye may transmit pressure and dislodge the contact lens. Consider placing a loose suture at the end of surgery to secure the free cap.

Do not proceed with laser ablation if the cap diameter is smaller than the optical zone.

If a free cap cannot be retrieved, the excimer laser treatment should be aborted and retreatment deferred until refractive stability is achieved.

PEARL #17: FLAP BUTTONHOLES

Of all flap complications, buttonholes are the most disconcerting to the surgeon. Most of the time, recognized risk factors are not present, and measures to reduce the incidence of this complication are often elusive.

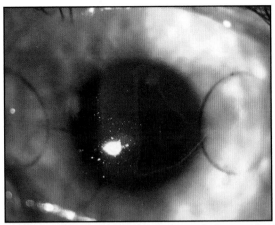 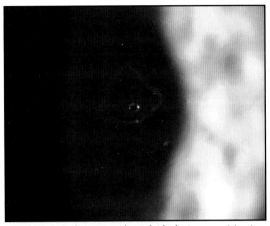

Figure 4-2 (Pearl 17). The LASIK buttonhole triangle sign. Gientian violet corneal marks help in repositioning the flap in the appropriate position, minimizing the risk of flap folds and epithelial ingrowth.

Thin, irregular, and perforated flaps seem to result from a common etiology: inadequate coupling of the blade to the cornea. Buttonholes occur when a dimple in the cornea is missed by the blade and remains uncut. Many etiologies have been suggested for the occurrence of this phenomenon. Steep corneas have been compared to tennis balls that buckle centrally upon applanating pressure. Another possible explanation is that higher keratometric values offer increased resistance to cutting when applanated, leading to upward movement of the blade. The latter is probably more applicable to keratomes with lower oscillation rates. Poor blade quality has also been presented as an explanation, especially when a cluster of cases is encountered. In our experience, we suspect microsuction loss to be the main reason behind flap buttonholes. Inadequate suction may occur in cases of conjunctival incarceration in the suction port (pseudosuction) or simply from a poorly functioning vacuum unit.

We have noticed that LASIK buttonholes (with the Hansatome keratome) invariably have a triangular shape (Figure 4-2). Typically, the base of the triangle is facing away from the surgeon.

If a buttonhole is encountered (especially centrally), it is best to call off the procedure and reposition the flap without laser treatment. We also advise to abort the procedure in cases of "near buttonholes." In those cases, Bowman's layer is found uncut either centrally or in the peripheral cornea, but the epithelial remains grossly intact. We believe that these cases are prone to the same complications as full-thickness buttonholes and should be approached as such.

It has become obvious to many LASIK surgeons that recutting at a later date is not advisable in these situations due to the risk of double flaps. The latter is particularly true after the advent of Mitomycin C (MMC) as an adjunctive antiscarring agent with surface ablation. We have devised a treatment algorithm to follow when a flap buttonhole is encountered. The infiltration of epithelial cells through the buttonhole determines which course of action is best to take. After a buttonhole, two scenarios present themselves in the first few days:

Scenario 1 (Figure 4-3): An epithelial ingrowth is present at the edge of the buttonhole. A higher index of suspicion for epithelial ingrowth around the margins of a buttonhole should be maintained in the early period after its occurrence. This can be a devastating complication because central stromal melting may ensue. Immediate intervention is warranted in these cases. We recommend a staged approach. The goal of the first stage is essentially therapeutic and is intended to obliterate the infiltrated epithelial cells. An initial 6.5-mm phototherapeutic keratectomy (PTK) treatment is applied at a depth of 40 to 50 μm. Ten-micron increments are then applied with slit lamp examination in between until the ingrowth is satisfactorily ablated. If the total amount of laser pulses applied in the first stage exceeds 50 μm, the refractive treatment is delayed to a later stage after a new stable refraction is obtained. At that time, surface ablation is repeated to correct the remaining refractive error. This approach avoids the risk of a hyperopic result if the full refractive treatment is applied on top of a significant PTK ablation.

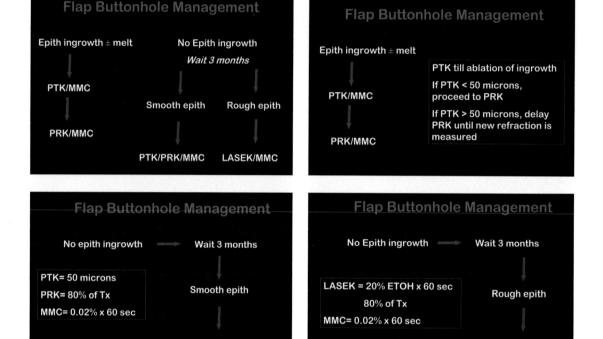

Figure 4-3 (Pearl 17). LASIK buttonhole management algorithm.

Scenario 2 (Figure 4-3): No epithelial ingrowth is noted at the edge of the buttonhole. In this situation, it is best to wait at least 3 months before deciding on further action. If the epithelium is smooth at that time, it is used as a masking agent during a PTK/PRK ablation. Using "black stromal appearance" as a guide to complete epithelial ablation is not as easy as in virgin corneas due to epithelial irregularity. Another approach is to apply a standard 40- to 50-µm PTK treatment followed by the refractive ablation. The irregularity in epithelial thickness may result in overcorrection with either approach. Therefore, we advise reducing the refractive laser treatment by 20%. Figure 4-4 shows a LASIK buttonhole before and after PRK/PTK treatment.

If after 3 months the epithelial surface is more irregular than the underlying buttonholed stroma, it is better to remove it with 20% alcohol applied for 60 seconds. The alcohol time is critical to avoid adherence of the epithelium to the edges of the hole and disrupt it during peeling. Similarly, we avoid recutting with the Intralase due to the manipulation needed to lift the flap.

We recommend 60 seconds of MMC application to prevent central scarring in a buttonhole situation. By following the above protocol, we have obtained excellent results in patients with buttonholed flaps. Such an approach ensures no loss of BCVA in the majority of cases.

The incidence of perforated flaps (as well as thin and irregular ones) may be reduced if the surgeon ensures adequate suction, inspects the blades, adjusts the keratome plate thickness settings according to corneal curvature, and ensures adequate IOP before cutting the flap. Accurate IOP measurement may be achieved by using a pneumotonometer. Care should be taken to avoid conjunctival clogging in the suction port, which could lead to a discrepancy between the IOP and the suction pressure recorded on the microkeratome vacuum console.

Inspection of the microkeratome blade under the operating microscope before engaging it in the suction ring is helpful to rule out manufacturing or other preoperative damage to the blade. It is best to keep the microkeratome away from hard surfaces after assembly in order to avoid subsequent blade damage.

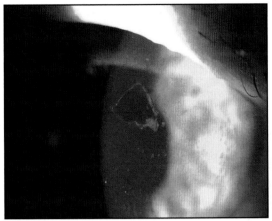 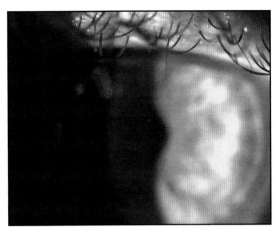

Figure 4-4 (Pearl 17). LASIK buttonhole before and after PTK/PRK treatment.

Table 4-1
SITUATIONS BEST MANAGED BY ABORTING THE LASIK PROCEDURE
• Poor suction despite corrective measures
• Flap smaller than the intended optical zone
• Flap with hinge within the optical zone
• Buttonholes and near-buttonholes
• Irregular flaps

Always Remember...

The safest way to proceed when a thin, irregular, or buttonholed flap is encountered may be to reposition the flap and abort the procedure.

IOP above 80 mm Hg may be essential for safer flap creation.

PEARL #18: THE ABORTED LASIK AND THE REPEAT LASIK

There comes a time in every surgical procedure when leaving the surgical field is the lesser of two (or more) evils. When is it best to reposition the flap, abandon the procedure, and possibly attempt the procedure at a later time (Table 4-1)?

Obtaining adequate suction in certain globes is occasionally an elusive target. This may occur in small hyperopic eyes, flat or small diameter corneas, and narrow palpebral fissures. If the level of myopia permits, one has to remember that PRK is always an available option, and patients must be made aware of this alternative and give consent prior to the procedure. A surgeon might be tempted to extend an incomplete flap with a crescent blade or similar instrument (see Figure 4-1). This might lead to flap truncation, perforation, or an uneven stromal bed and scarring. Understandably, the closer the hinge is to the visual axis, the riskier this maneuver will be. If the bed is large enough (not more than 0.5 mm of unexposed stroma at the hinge), laser treatment may be possible (with adequate protection to the underside of the flap).

An irregular flap indicates an irregular stromal bed and is best allowed to heal in position to avoid the risk of inducing irregular astigmatism (Figure 4-5).

Figure 4-5 (Pearl 18). Irregular flap: the corneal light reflex is valuable to detect an irregular flap and stromal bed. This complication is mostly associated with blade defects or suction loss. The flap should be repositioned and treatment performed at a later date.

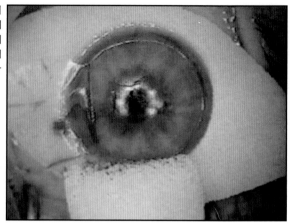

Figure 4-6 (Pearl 18). Flap lift technique using ring Forceps. Jeweler's forceps can be used to lift the edge of the LASIK flap. Ring forceps are then used to lift the rest of the flap in a flap-rhexis fashion.

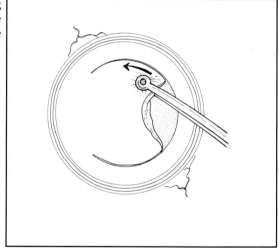

If a buttonhole or a near-buttonhole occurs, abortion of the LASIK procedure is preferable. Immediate laser ablation of the central epithelium by scraping or by the laser may lead to uneven ablation and loss of BCVA (see Pearl 17 for further discussion of buttonhole management).

Lifting LASIK corneal flaps can be accomplished several years after the initial procedure. Several flap problems can occur at the time of or shortly after enhancement:
- Tearing of the flap.
- Epithelial defects.
- Epithelial implantation and ingrowth.
- Flap folds.

Epithelial defects are associated with increased risk of ingrowth and with postoperative pain. The following technique may minimize the occurrence of these complications. The flap edge is identified at the slit lamp and marked with a marking pen. A 25-gauge needle or a Sinskey hook is used to lift the flap edge either temporally or inferiorly. The patient is then positioned at the laser, and forceps are used to lift the flap. Gentle peeling is performed in a flap-rhexis fashion along the flap edge to avoid lifting the surrounding epithelium (Figure 4-6). Epithelial tags are noted quite often as extending over the stromal edge after flap lifting. These should be gently positioned away from the area of laser ablation and draped over the flap at the end of the procedure.

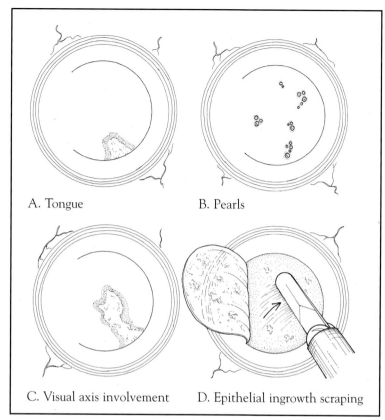

A. Tongue   B. Pearls

C. Visual axis involvement   D. Epithelial ingrowth scraping

Figure 4-7 (Pearl 19). Epithelial ingrowth patterns and method of removal. Thorough scraping of both the stromal bed and the underside of the flap must be performed.

Flap folds are more likely to occur after enhancement in part due to additional laser ablation of the central stroma with a tenting effect of the overlying flap. Adequate repositioning according to preplaced corneal marking and even applanating pressure should lead to a smooth flap surface.

Always Remember...

Epithelial defects will increase the chance of epithelial ingrowth due to a high mitotic activity after the injury.

PEARL #19: EPITHELIAL INGROWTH: LEAVE OR LIFT?

Epithelium under the corneal flap can cause induced hyperopia and irregular astigmatism secondary to stromal melting. Swift intervention is sometimes needed to prevent these complications.

If the epithelium is noted to progress toward the visual axis or if a significant hyperopic shift or loss of BCVA is encountered, lifting of the flap and scraping of the epithelium should be performed promptly. Scraping can be performed with a blunt spatula or a #69 blade (Figure 4-7). It is important to remember to scrape the stromal bed as well as the stromal aspect of the flap. The Melki LASIK Flap Suction Stabilizer (Rhein Medical, Tampa, Fla, no financial interest) can provide a solid surface to allow adequate and thorough epithelial scraping (Figure 4-8). The same instruments can also be used to flatten flap folds. Flap folds connected to the peripheral epithelium may provide a conduit for epithelial cell infiltration. Similarly, an epithelial defect adjacent to the edge of the flap should be followed closely due to the presence of high epithelial mitotic activity. Fluorescein staining often reveals a pinpoint area with an open fistula where cells are infiltrating under the flap.

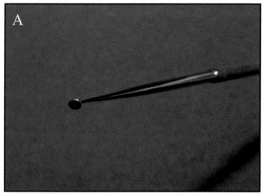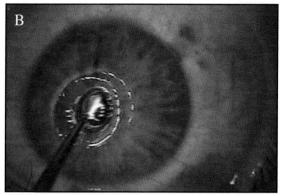

Figure 4-8 (Pearl 19). The Pineda iron for management of flap folds. (A) The instrument is designed as an iron with a flat undersurface and rounded edges to avoid epithelial injury and (B) is used to gently massage the flap either at the slit lamp or under the operating microscope. (Courtesy of Roberto Pineda II, MD, Massachusetts Eye and Ear Infirmary.)

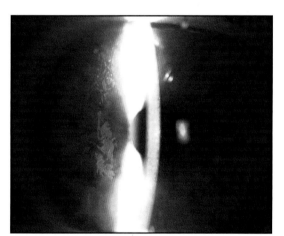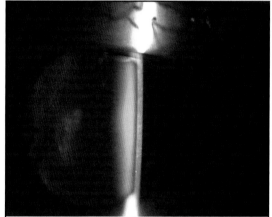

Figure 4-9 (Pearl 19). Recurrent epithelial ingrowth infiltrating from the superior aspect of the flap.

Small isolated epithelial pearls are usually self-limited and do not progress. Epithelial tongues connected to the flap edge are more worrisome; they need to be scraped if they exhibit a rapid rate of progression or if they threaten the visual axis (Figure 4-9).

Recurrent epithelial ingrowth may require suturing of the flap. We usually apply at least three interrupted sutures straddling the edge of the flap in the area of the ingrowth (Figure 4-10). Interrupted sutures need to be placed around the flap circumference to ensure even stretching. Flap sutures are typically removed 3 to 4 weeks later. We prefer removing two sutures at a time with topical steroid coverage to avoid the risk of DLK. A stable, untreated epithelial ingrowth will end up scarring down with occasional innocuous melting at the flap edge (Figure 4-11).

Always Remember...

The leading edge of an epithelial ingrowth may be more extensive than recognized at the slit lamp. A high index of suspicion must be maintained.

Recalcitrant flap edema may be due to underlying epithelial ingrowth.

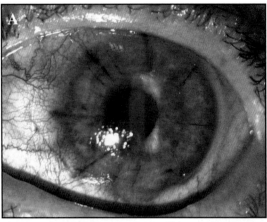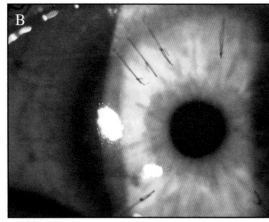

Figure 4-10 (Pearls 19 and 20). Flap suturing for recurrent epithelial ingrowth.

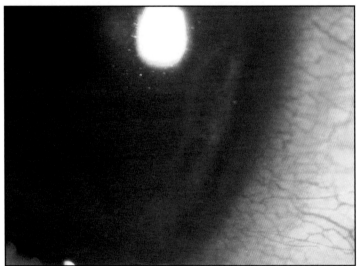

Figure 4-11 (Pearl 19). Flap edge scarring after spontaneous epithelial ingrowth resolution.

PEARL #20: FLATTENING THE RECALCITRANT LASIK FLAP FOLD

Flap folds can induce irregular astigmatism and loss of BCVA, especially if they involve the visual axis. Macrofolds are easily seen by slit lamp examination and represent full-thickness flap folding in a linear fashion. On the other hand, microfolds may represent wrinkles in Bowman's layer or in the epithelial basement membrane. They are best seen as negative staining lines with sodium fluorescein. The incidence of folds requiring intervention ranges between 0.2% and 1.5%.

Flap folds result from uneven alignment of the flap edge and the peripheral epithelium. This can occur in the setting of an unequally hydrated stromal bed prior to flap repositioning. Thinner and larger flaps tend to shift more readily with resultant surface wrinkling. Uneven sponge smoothing maneuvers can result in radial (with centrifugal movement) or circumferential folds (with centripetal movement). A higher incidence of flap folds occurs in higher myopes. This is due to the reduced central convexity and stromal support, resulting in flap redundancy that may be difficult to flatten.

Management options include simple lifting and refloating of the flap, ironing of the flap, epithelial scraping, and placement of sutures to stretch the flap in position. Probst and Machat described a technique using the red reflex as a way to better detect flap wrinkles during flattening procedures. Smoothing of the flap is best achieved by even distribution of the forces applied to the flap surface. This can be performed with nonfragmenting sponges or their equivalent. Instruments such as the Pineda corneal LASIK

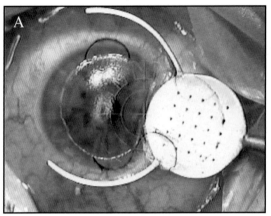
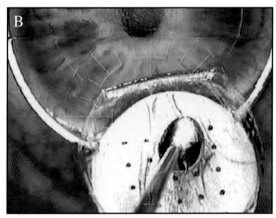

Figure 4-12 (Pearl 20). (A) The Melki LASIK Flap Suction Stabilizer. (B) This instrument can be used to stabilize the flap to facilitate scraping epithelial cells from the underside of the flap or flattening flap folds.

iron (Asico, Westmont, Ill) (see Figure 4-8A) can also be used to flatten isolated flaps at the slit lamp or under the operating microscope by gently pressing on them (see Figure 4-8B). The Melki flap stabilizer (Figure 4-12A) was designed to facilitate flap fold flattening from the stromal side. A Pineda iron can be used in combination to help with that task (Figure 4-12B). Other reported strategies include hydrating the flap with hypotonic saline (60% to 80%), which may facilitate leveling of the flap surface.

Fixed folds are sometimes encountered and probably occur when epithelial hyperplasia has time to form in the crevices formed by the folds. Epithelial debridement over the wrinkled area may relieve contractures that occur secondary to the presumed epithelial hyperplasia in these longer-standing folds. Recalcitrant wrinkling may respond to placement of 10-0 or 11-0 nylon sutures.

Always Remember…

The earlier a flap is attended to, the higher the chances of fold flattening.

PEARL # 21: LASIK FLAPS: IS LARGER BETTER?

Microkeratomes offer the possibility to choose the size of the corneal flap during LASIK. The range usually extends from 8.5 to 10 mm in diameter. Smaller flaps may lead to an increase in postsurgical complications when compared to larger flaps. When creating a flap of any size, the surgeon must remember that steeper corneas lead to larger than intended flaps and flatter corneas lead to smaller than intended flaps.

Large flaps provide large ablation zones for the treatment of overcorrections.

LASIK treatment for myopia requires an ablation zone 6 to 6.5 mm in diameter. Unfortunately, the correction of myopia sometimes leads to an overcorrection, which requires an ablation zone of 9.0 mm. If a larger flap has been cut, the flap can simply be lifted and the corneal stroma ablated to adjust the refractive error.

If the original LASIK surgery was performed with a smaller flap, however, the available ablation zone may be less than ideal. Recutting with a 9.5-mm ring is not advisable at this point because it may lead to double flaps that induce irregular astigmatism. Ablation using the small flap is also not satisfactory because the ablation of the surrounding epithelium may lead to an increase in the risk of epithelium ingrowth. If the stromal area is too small for proper hyperopic treatment, a protective lubricant gel can be applied to the edges of the cut flap to protect it from laser treatment, and then ablate as usual. Because most hyperopic treatment occurs within the mid-periphery of the eye, well within the 8-mm zone, this decrease in the ablation area will minimally diminish the effectiveness of the hyperopic treatment.

Larger flaps are more adherent to the underlying cornea. This is readily noted when lifting flaps during enhancements. The edges of larger LASIK flaps lie closer to the richly vascularized corneal limbus at the edge of the eye and adhere strongly in this region. The reports of flap dislocations caused by physical trauma several months following LASIK suggest the importance of improved flap adhesions. A large flap would help to minimize the risk of such dislocations.

Larger LASIK flaps are more protective of the visual axis. This is illustrated in situations such as DLK, epithelial ingrowth, or other conditions necessitating flap suturing.

DLK is an inflammatory condition with multivariate etiology that starts at the LASIK flap edge. The inflammation then spreads towards the visual axis and may lead, in severe cases, to corneal melting and scarring. A larger flap would move the site of the onset of inflammation further from the visual axis, giving the surgeon more time to intervene.

Epithelial cells can implant in the interface due to seeding during surgery or due to migration under the flap. Epithelial ingrowth extending from the edge of the flap is a more serious complication. A continual source of epithelial cells is supplied to the ingrowth by the peripheral epithelial, usually through a microfistula, leading to progressive ingrowth that can cause central corneal melting and scarring and loss of vision. The creation of a larger LASIK flap would place the edge of the flap further from the visual axis and give the surgeon more time to observe and intervene.

Flap decentration can occur secondary to incorrect positioning of the suction ring or because of globe movement (oozing), even after the suction has been applied. The latter is more common in patients with larger corneas. Corneal oozing can continue throughout the procedure and can lead to significant flap decentration. A small, decentered flap is more likely to cause visual damage than a large flap because the edge of the flap will likely lie closer to the visual axis. A combination of scarring at the edge of the flap and a large mesopic pupil may lead to significant visual aberration at night. A larger flap would place the edge of the flap further from the edge of the visual axis and be more forgiving in decentered cases.

Flap suturing may be needed to correct LASIK complications such as recurrent epithelial ingrowth or persistent corneal folds. The sutures are usually placed radially at the edge of the flap at approximately 50% corneal thickness (see Figure 4-10B). The suturing of a smaller flap places the stitches closer to the pupillary edge than a larger flap, which may lead to astigmatism and possibly persistent aberrations. The additional risk of surrounding inflammation or infection due to sutures supports the benefit of placing them in the most peripheral cornea.

Smaller LASIK flaps may offer some advantages, such as a deceased incidence of dry eyes due to a reduced injury to the corneal nerves. Another purported advantage is lesser risk of corneal ectasia due to a smaller area of corneal compromise. There are no definitive studies proving these advantages.

Always Remember....

Larger flaps displace some LASIK complications and their treatment towards the periphery, hence protecting the visual axis.

BIBLIOGRAPHY

Durrie DS, Aziz AA. Lift-flap retreatment after laser in situ keratomileusis. *J Refract Surg.* 1999;15:150-153.

Farah SG, Azar DT, Gurdal C, et al. Laser in situ keratomileusis: literature review of a developing technique. *J Cataract Refract Surg.* 1998;24:989-1006.

Gimbel HV, Penno EE, van Westenbrugge JA, et al. Incidence and management of intraoperative and early postoperative complications in 1000 consecutive laser in situ keratomileusis cases. *Ophthalmology.* 1998;105:1839-1847; discussion 1847-1848.

Helena MC, Meisler D, Wilson SE. Epithelial growth within the lamellar interface after laser in situ keratomileusis (LASIK) [see comments]. *Cornea.* 1997;16:300-305.

Holland SP, Srivannaboon S, Reinstein DZ. Avoiding serious corneal complications of laser assisted in situ keratomileusis and photorefractive keratectomy. *Ophthalmology.* 2000;107(4):640-652.

Kapadia MS, Wilson SE. Transepithelial photorefractive keratectomy for treatment of thin flaps or caps after complicated laser in situ keratomileusis. *Am J Ophthalmol.* 1998;126:827-829.

Leung AT, Rao SK, Cheng AC, Yu EW, Fan DS, Lam DS. Pathogenesis and management of laser in situ keratomileusis flap but-tonhole. *J Cataract Refract Surg.* 2000;26(3):358-362.

Melki SA, Azar DT. LASIK complications: etiology, management, and prevention. *Surv Ophthalmol.* 2001;46(2):95-116.

Melki SA, Nguyen A, Gatinel D. *The LASIK buttonhole and the Bermuda triangle.* Video. San Diego, Calif: ASCRS; 2004.

Melki SA, Proano CE, Azar DT. Optical disturbances and their management after myopic laser in situ keratomileusis. *Int Ophthalmol Clin.* 2000;40(1):45-56.

Probst LE, Machat J. Removal of flap striae following laser in situ keratomileusis. *J Cataract Refract Surg.* 1998;24:153-155.

Shah MN, Misra M, Wihelmus KR, Koch DD. Diffuse lamellar keratitis associated with epithelial defects after laser in situ keratomileusis. *J Cataract Refract Surg.* 2000;26(9):1312-1318.

Tham VM, Maloney RK. Microkeratome complications of laser in situ keratomileusis. *Ophthalmology.* 2000;107(5):920-924.

Updegraff SA, Kritzinger MS. Laser in situ keratomileusis technique. *Curr Opin Ophthalmol.* 2000;11(4):267-272.

Von Kulajta P, Stark WJ, O'Brien TP. Management of flap striae. *Int Ophthalmol Clin.* 2000;40(3):87-92.

Walker MB, Wilson SE. Incidence and prevention of epithelial growth within the interface after laser in situ keratomileusis. *Cornea.* 2000;19(2):170-173.

Wang MY, Maloney RK. Epithelial ingrowth after laser in situ keratomileusis. *Am J Ophthalmol.* 2000;129(6):746-751.

CHAPTER 5

FOUR
PHOTOREFRACTIVE KERATECTOMY, LASEK, AND EPI-LASIK PEARLS

Eric J. Dudenhoefer, MD and Dimitri T. Azar, MD

This chapter addresses issues relevant to PRK. Excimer laser PRK remains a viable treatment for the correction of low to moderate myopia and in situations where lamellar or other refractive surgical procedures may be problematic.

PEARL #22: METHODS OF EPITHELIAL DEBRIDEMENT IN PHOTOREFRACTIVE KERATECTOMY

Epithelial removal before PRK allows for application of excimer laser energy directly on Bowman's membrane and the stroma. It has been proposed that the ideal method of de-epithelialization prior to PRK should be atraumatic, result in rapid debridement, and produce a small epithelial defect with sharp edges. Our preference is to use diluted ethanol; however, other methods of epithelial debridement have been used successfully, including mechanical scraping with a dull or sharp blade, powered rotary brushes, laser scraping, and transepithelial ablation.

Each method has its associated drawbacks. Mechanical removal is performed using a dull spatula or sharp blade to centripetally remove a previously demarcated zone of central epithelium. This may leave islands of retained epithelium and ridges and irregularities in Bowman's layer, respectively. Time for completion of epithelial removal can also be prolonged, especially for inexperienced surgeons, introducing the problem of variability of stromal dehydration and possible alteration in treatment effect.

Epithelial removal using a rotating plastic brush attached to a motor unit appears simple, fast, and easy and is reported to leave a clean, clear Bowman's layer. However, this technique may result in eye wandering and a larger zone of epithelial removal due to obstruction of the visual axis.

Transepithelial laser and laser-scrape have also been utilized successfully. In the former, the laser is used as the sole means of epithelial removal. The surgeon typically sets the laser for an assumed epithelial depth of 50 μm or uses the visible decrease in fluorescence that occurs when the laser completes the epithelial ablation and enters stroma as the guides for treatment. However, there is a tendency toward overtreatment with this technique, which must be taken into consideration when determining the ablation parameters.

With the laser scrape method, the laser is set for a depth of 40 μm. Then, the surgeon resorts to a scraping technique for final epithelial removal. This is often faster than mechanical removal but reintroduces some of the risks of mechanical removal mentioned above. In addition, increased patient anxiety from prolonged exposure to the loud sound of the laser pulses, increased wear and tear on the laser optics, and increased use of gasses may be minor drawbacks of this technique.

In view of the above, we prefer to use 18% ethanol applied for 25 seconds as our method of epithelial removal. Ethanol treatment for epithelial dissection has a well-documented history of safety and efficacy and avoids the drawbacks of mechanical and laser epithelial removal techniques. Namely, it avoids the ragged edges, larger-than-intended de-epithelialized zones, retained islands of epithelium, defects in Bowman's layer common to mechanical techniques, and the minor drawbacks of optics wear and increased use of gasses with the laser methods. This technique is illustrated in Figure 5-1.

Figure 5-1 (Pearl 22). Alcohol-assisted de-epithelialization. (A) The area for epithelial removal is delineated by firmly placing a 7-mm optical zone marker upon the cornea, centered on the pupil. Two drops of 18% ethanol are placed inside the reservoir (the walls of the marker should be at least 3 mm high). (B) After 25 seconds, a cellulose sponge is used to completely absorb the ethanol. A slight rotating downward pressure prior to removing the optical zone marker will separate the ethanol-treated epithelium from the untreated peripheral rim. (C) The loosened epithelium is removed with another dry cellulose sponge. It usually comes off as a single sheet. (D) "Microcoat" any surface

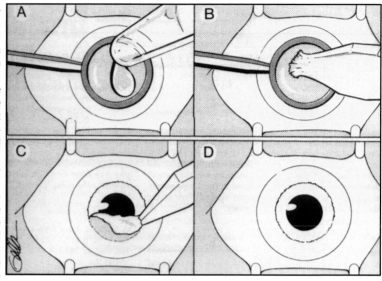

irregularities by passing another cellulose sponge moistened with 0.5% methylcellulose (eg, Refresh [Allergen, Irvine, Calif]) across the corneal surface. Dry any excess fluid. The surface is now ready for the laser ablation. (Reprinted with permission from Elsevier Science. Abad JC, An B, Power W, et al. A prospective evaluation of alcohol assisted versus mechanical epithelial removal before photorefractive keratectomy. *Ophthalmology*. 1997;104(10):1568.)

Always Remember...

Epithelial removal for a retreatment may require longer than 25 seconds of exposure to ethanol to overcome a more adherent hyperplastic epithelium.

PEARL #23: LASEK AND EPI-LASIK

The major limitations of PRK are subepithelial haze, postoperative pain, and prolonged visual rehabilitation brought about by epithelial removal. In an attempt to circumvent these problems, these surgical techniques have been developed. Epithelial coverage is restored immediately through creation of a hinged epithelial flap, which is lifted at the beginning of surgery and replaced after ablation. In LASEK, epithelial "Flap PRK" is performed using 18% ethanol. In Epi-LASIK, the epithelial flap is performed using a modified microkeratome. These techniques appear more reproducible than standard PRK and may offer faster re-epithelialization, reduced postoperative pain, and shorter visual rehabilitation time.

Patients receive topical broad-spectrum antibiotics in the eye to be treated 30 minutes before surgery. A sterile drape is placed around the eye after which topical anesthetic drops are instilled and a lid speculum is applied. The LASEK technique is described and illustrated in Figure 5-2.

Overlapping circular marks are preplaced on the cornea to facilitate later epithelial realignment. Ethanol (18%) is placed into the reservoir of a 7-mm semi-sharp marker. The ethanol is left in place as described previously, and then absorbed with a dry sponge to avoid peripheral corneal exposure.

One arm of a Vannas forceps is used to demarcate and lift the edge of the epithelium. Using a dry nonfragmenting sponge, the loosened epithelium is peeled as a single sheet, leaving a flap of epithelium with a hinge still attached.

In Epi-LASIK, an epithelial separator is used to create the epithelial sheet. Laser ablation of the exposed Bowman's layer and stroma is then performed. The epithelial flap, generated chemically or mechanically, is repositioned on the stromal bed. Using great care, the wound edges are realigned using the preplaced marks as a guide while avoiding epithelial defects. After waiting several minutes for

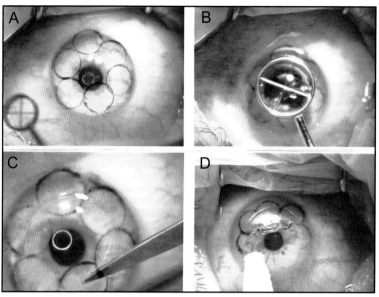

Figure 5-2 (Pearl 23). The LASEK technique: (A) gentian violet fiducial marks are applied to the cornea; (B) alcohol-assisted de-epithelialization is performed. The epithelium is peeled as a single sheet using (C) a blunt metal instrument or (D) a Murocel sponge.

epithelial adhesion to occur, topical diclofenac sodium 0.1%, ciprofloxacin, and fluorometholone 0.1% are placed upon the eye followed by placement of a bandage soft contact lens and removal of the lid speculum.

Postoperative care consists of oral narcotics as needed (prn), a topical fluoroquinolone four times a day (qid), and prednisolone acetate 1% qid for 2 weeks. The bandage contact lens is removed when any necessary re-epithelialization is complete (day 1 to 3).

Always Remember...

Apply gentle but firm pressure to the corneal trephine during ethanol application to ensure the alcohol reaches the subepithelial dissection plane.

Take care to avoid ethanol exposure outside the marker reservoir. If this occurs secondary to sudden eye movement, the eye is washed with balanced salt solution with no adverse consequences.

PEARL #24: HANDLING HAZE AND DECENTRATION IN SURFACE ABLATION

Corneal subepithelial haze is commonly seen as part of the normal corneal healing response following PRK (Figure 5-3). This subepithelial scarring of the cornea peaks at 3 to 6 months following PRK with a steady decrease in severity until 18 months postoperatively. The degree of haze varies among individual patients, yet presents with greater density and frequency as the degree of intended correction increases. Haze is associated with loss of BCVA, regression of treatment effect, decreased CS, and light scatter around bright light sources, especially at night.

Postoperative treatment with topical corticosteroids appears to reduce the severity of post-PRK haze. Despite this prophylaxis, however, some patients may still develop persistent, visually significant haze. Topical steroids and superficial keratectomy have successfully improved corneal clarity and significantly reversed associated refractive regression, but the effect is often transient, requiring chronic or repeated treatments with the associated well-described complications.

The use of the antimetabolite MMC following epithelial debridement has been shown to be effective in restoring corneal clarity and reversing regression in patients with significant subepithelial fibrosis that recurs after surgical debridement and steroids. Its safety profile has been established, in part, through

Figure 5-3 (Pearl 24). Corneal haze after PRK.

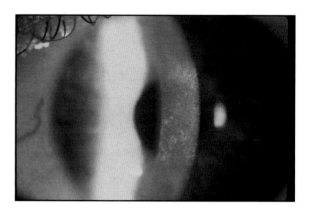

routine use in glaucoma filtering surgery, pterygium excision, and the treatment of conjunctival and corneal intraepithelial neoplasia. Despite limited toxicity in these treatments, however, rare reports have emerged describing corneoscleral melts after even a single application of MMC 0.02% for 3 minutes during pterygium surgery. Accordingly, care should be exercised with its use, especially in individuals with a history of ocular surface disease (ie, keratoconjunctivitis sicca and ocular rosacea). The recommended regimen described by Majmudar et al is as follows:

- Instill topical anesthetic.
- Remove the corneal epithelium with a #64 Beaver blade (or other), and gently, mechanically remove as much fibrosis as possible.
- Place a sterile 6-mm circular sponge soaked in MMC (0.02%) on the corneal surface for 2 minutes. Limit MMC exposure to the central 6 mm of the cornea.
- Remove the sponge, and irrigate the ocular surface liberally with BSS (Alcon Surgical, Fort Worth, Tex).
- Cover the eye with antibiotic-steroid ointment, and place either a patch or bandage contact lens (based on practice preference).

Recent reports suggest that use of more dilute MMC for shorter durations may be useful for prevention of subepithelial haze in higher myopes.

After epithelial debridement, a low dose of MMC (0.02% = 0.2 mg/ml) for a short duration (2 minutes) can be effective in combating persistent, visually significant haze and regression. This should be considered in patients who do not respond to steroid treatment.

When PRK haze coexists with a loss of BCVA, a hard contact lens over-refraction will determine the relative contribution of irregular astigmatism versus corneal scarring.

Always Remember...

PRK in moderately high myopes should be avoided whenever possible to prevent haze. Other surgical alternatives, including LASIK, should be considered in these patients.

As in other keratorefractive surgical procedures, maintaining centration of laser treatment in relation to the entrance pupil throughout PRK is essential for achieving best visual outcomes. Treatment decentration may be associated with reduced visual function due to glare, edge effects, and refractive errors.

Treatment displacement (shift) is caused by initial lack of centration that is not rectified or from involuntary eye movement during the procedure (also not corrected), ultimately resulting in an off-center treatment (Figure 5-4). Intraoperative drift occurs when the eye wanders involuntarily during surgery, and the decentration is corrected while ablation continues or when the surgeon recognizes and attempts to correct initial decentration during treatment.

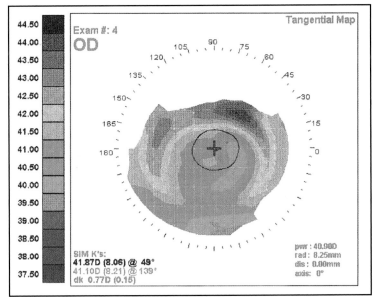

Figure 5-4 (Pearl 24). Tangential topographic analysis of a right eye 1 month after PRK (showing high inferotemporal displacement of laser treatment zone r = 0.81 mm). Visual acuity of 20/20 was achieved. The black circle and black cross on the map represent the pupillary margin and the position of the pupillary center, respectively. (Reprinted with permission from Elsevier Science. Azar DT, Yeh PC. Corneal topographic evaluation of decentration in photorefractive keratectomy: treatment displacement vs intraoperative drift. *Am J Ophthamol.* 1997;124(3):312-320.)

Drift results in a less uniform distribution of surface powers within the treatment zone and irregular astigmatism. The degree of intraoperative drift has been shown to correlate highly with reduction of BCVA following PRK.

Displacement without intraoperative drift may occur if a tracker is used when the surgeon is unaware of the decentration or is aware but chooses not to correct it. It results in a more uniform ablation zone and does not appear to lead to a significant reduction in BCVA.

Accordingly, when treatment has begun and the surgeon recognizes that the treatment was decentered from the outset, the accepted conventional approach of recentering the treatment, which is aimed at reducing the problem of edge effects, may lead to worse quality of vision and possible loss of BCVA (drift effect). Maintaining the initial alignment throughout the procedure, which ensures a more uniform ablation zone, will maximize visual acuity.

During initially centered treatment, however, involuntary micro- and macro-saccades may occur. In most instances, the surgeon is able to maintain centration by tracking and adjusting for micromovements of the eye even if no tracker is used. However, if the surgeon is unable to maintain centration during laser ablation (macro-saccade), the eye should not be repositioned while ablation continues. In this situation, ablation should be discontinued immediately, the initial alignment re-established, and treatment continued. Following these guidelines will maximize the uniformity of the ablation zone and give the best possible postoperative visual result.

Always Remember…

Avoiding the urge to recenter initial displacement (present at the onset of ablation) may maximize postoperative BCVA.

Pearl #25: Photorefractive Keratectomy for Residual Myopia After Radial Keratotomy

Until recent years, RK was among the most widely used surgical techniques to correct myopia. Given the procedure's propensity for hyperopic drift during the postoperative period (43% progression of +1.00 D from 1 to 10 years postoperatively [PERK Study]), "conservative RK" has been widely advocated, leaving patients with intentional undercorrections initially. However, significant undercorrections occur and persist in some cases. Therapeutic strategies to consider for correction of residual myopia one year after RK include spectacles, contact lenses, and reoperations. The surgical options include redeepening the incisions, extending existing RK incisions centripetally or centrifugally, placing additional RK incisions, or performing another keratorefractive procedure such as excimer laser PRK or LASIK.

In RK, radial incisions flex the peripheral cornea, leading to flattening of the central cornea. The amount of central flattening that can be achieved using this technique, however, is limited. Excimer laser PRK and LASIK present attractive alternatives to placement of multiple incisions or extensive RK because they act by a different mechanism. Central corneal flattening is achieved via direct ablation with the laser.

We believe that, in many cases, LASIK may be the procedure of choice to correct post-RK refractive errors due to the reduced incidence of subepithelial haze and better predictability of the final refractive error. However, in cases where the LASIK procedure poses a high risk (ie, patients with epithelial plugs or thin corneas), PRK may be a viable alternative.

Both the original pre-RK refractive error as well as the degree of residual pre-PRK (post-RK) refractive error affect the outcome of PRK after RK. The PRK after RK Study Group showed that the most predictable refractive outcomes and least amount of subepithelial haze were achieved in eyes with original refractive errors (pre-RK) of <6.00 D and residual errors of <3.00 D. Although some regression of the refractive correction can still be expected in the first postoperative year, the procedure tends to be most predictable and stable for patients with lower refractive errors.

We do not recommend PRK to correct residual myopia after RK for patients with high degrees of original pre-RK and of residual pre-PRK myopia.

Always Remember…

Consider ethanol epithelial removal or transepithelial ablation to prevent RK incision dehiscence from scraping techniques. This approach may reduce subepithelial scarring by reducing keratocyte activation.

Consider PRK for treatment of residual myopia one year or more after RK for patients with unstable RK incisions, pre-RK refractions of <6.00 D, and residual refractive errors of <3.00 D. For higher refractive errors, consider LASIK initially.

BIBLIOGRAPHY

Abad JC, An B, Power W, et al. A prospective evaluation of alcohol-assisted versus mechanical epithelial removal before photorefractive keratectomy. *Ophthalmology.* 1997;104:1566-1573.

Azar DT, Ang RT, Lee JB, et al. Laser subepithelial keratomileusis: electron microscopy and visual outcomes of flap photorefractive keratectomy. *Curr Opin Ophthalmol.* 2001;12(4):323-328. Review.

Azar DT, Tuli S, Benson RA, Hardten DR, PRK after RK Study Group. Photorefractive keratectomy for residual myopia after radial keratotomy. *J Cataract Refract Surg.* 1998;24:303-311.

Azar DT, Yeh PC. Corneal topographic evaluation of decentration in photorefractive keratectomy: treatment displacement vs. intraoperative drift. *Am J Ophthalmol.* 1997;124:312-320.

Campos M, Hertzog L, Wang XW, et al. Corneal surface after de-epithelialization using a sharp and a dull instrument. *Ophthalmic Surg.* 1992;23:618-621.

Carones F, Fiore T, Brancato R. Mechanical vs. alcohol epithelial removal during photorefractive keratectomy. *J Refract Surg.* 1999;15:556-562.

Dougherty PJ, Hardten DR, Lindstrom RL. Corneoscleral melt after pterygium surgery using a single intraoperative application of Mitomycin C. *Cornea.* 1996;15:537-540.

Garty DS, Kerr Muir MG, Marshall J. Excimer laser photorefractive keratectomy: 18-month follow-up. *Ophthalmology.* 1992;99:1209-1219.

Gimbel HV, DeBroff BM, Beldows RA, et al. Comparison of laser and manual removal of corneal epithelium for photorefractive keratectomy. *J Refract Surg.* 1995;11:36-41.

Heigle TJ, Stulting RD, Palay DA. Treatment of recurrent conjunctival epithelial neoplasia with topical Mitomycin C. *Am J Ophthalmol.* 1997;124:397-399.

Mahar PS, Nwokora GE. Role of Mitomycin C in pterygium surgery. *Br J Ophthalmol.* 1993;77:433-435.

Majmudar PA, Forstot SL, Dennis RF, et al. Topical Mitomycin C for subepithelial fibrosis after refractive corneal surgery. *Ophthalmology.* 2000;107:89-94.

Pallikaris IG, Karoutis AD, Lydataki SE, Siganos DS. Rotating brush for fast removal of corneal epithelium. *J Refract Corneal Surg.* 1994;10:439-442.

Rubinfeld RS, Pfister RR, Stein RM, et al. Serious complications of topical Mitomycin C after pterygium surgery. *Ophthalmology.* 1992;99:1647-1654.

Shah S, Doyle SJ, Chatterjee A, et al. Comparison of 18% ethanol and mechanical debridement for epithelial removal before photorefractive keratectomy. *J Refract Surg.* 1998;14:212-214.

Shah SB, Lingua RW, Kim CH, Peters NT. Laser in situ keratomileusis to correct residual myopia and astigmatism after radial keratotomy. *J Cataract Refract Surg.* 2000;26:1152-1157.

Stein HA, Stein RM, Price C, Salim GA. Alcohol removal of the epithelium for excimer laser ablation: outcomes analysis. *J Cataract Refract Surg.* 1997;23:1160-1163.

Talamo JH, Gollamudi S, Green WR, et al. Modulation of corneal wound healing after excimer laser keratomileusis using topical Mitomycin C and steroids. *Arch Ophthalmol.* 1991;109:1141-1146.

Waring GO III, Lynn MJ, McDonnell PJ, PERK Study Group. Results of the prospective evaluation of radial keratotomy (PERK) study 10 years after surgery. *Arch Ophthalmol.* 1994;112:1298-1308.

Wong A, Yeh PC, Huong F, Azar D. Pathogenesis and management of haze after photorefractive keratectomy. *HK J Ophthalmol.* 1997;1:90-94.

CHAPTER 6

FOUR
PHOTOTHERAPEUTIC KERATECTOMY PEARLS

Shahzad Mian, MD and Dimitri T. Azar, MD

PTK with laser treatment is a useful tool that allows for effective removal of anterior corneal pathology and smoothing of surface irregularities. The submicron precision with which the depth and shape of laser ablative photodecompensation is controlled allows for a smooth surface for re-epithelialization and minimizes corneal scarring. The following review of criteria and techniques will aid in optimizing clinical results for PTK.

PEARL #26: LOCATION, LOCATION, LOCATION: DEPTH, DIAMETER, AND POSITION

A thorough preoperative evaluation to determine the depth, proximity to visual axis, and visual significance of the pathology is essential for optimizing visual outcomes. Results for PTK are best with depth of ablation less than 100 μm. Limiting ablation depth reduces large changes in the refractive state. PTK is effective for removal of pathology in Bowman's layer or in the anterior stroma (Figure 6-1). Despite the density of deeper stromal opacification, relatively superficial ablation (removing surface irregularities) contributes significantly to restoration of acuity. Estimation of the depth of the opacity can be approximated at the slit lamp with a narrow slit. The depth can be quantitated by using a modified Haag-Streit optical pachometer (Haag-Streit, Mason, Ohio). Alignment of the slit lamp and the microscope in relation to the corneal surface is used to obtain accurate measurements of pathology depth. Full-thickness corneal measurement is obtained by alignment of the endothelium of the upper field with epithelium of the lower field. Pachometry of the anterior corneal pathology is performed by aligning the posterior extent of the lesion with the epithelium of the lower field.

Evaluation of the proximity of the corneal opacity to the pupil is an important predictor of successful visual outcomes after PTK. Central corneal surface irregularities and opacities are good indications for PTK because treatment generally leads to a significant reduction in irregular astigmatism. Paracentral corneal pathology can also be visually significant, requiring treatment, but peripheral corneal opacities and surface irregularities are usually not visually significant. Anterior stromal scarring after pterygium removal consists of a paracentral, visually significant portion and a peripheral, visually insignificant portion. PTK is performed to smooth the paracentral changes, while the peripheral scar is ignored, typically requiring significantly less energy than when treating the peripheral portion. Treatment of peripheral lesions may, in fact, decrease final visual acuity because of induced irregular astigmatism from the PTK. Preoperative keratography can also be helpful in identifying visually significant peripheral opacities or irregularities.

Always Remember...

The depth of corneal pathology can be estimated at the slit lamp and can be quantitated by using an optical pachometer.

PTK should always be considered for visually significant pathology only. Treatment of visually insignificant areas should be avoided.

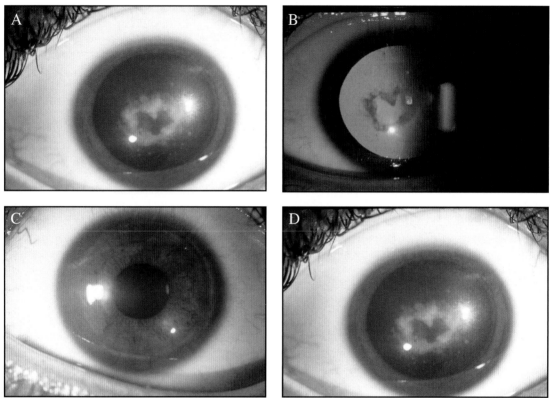

Figure 6-1 (Pearl 26). PTK in a patient with nonspecific familial anterior stromal dystrophy: (A, B) preoperative pictures and (C, D) postoperative pictures.

PEARL #27: BEST PREOPERATIVE REFRACTION FOR BETTER POSTOPERATIVE VISION

A complete preoperative evaluation includes documentation of uncorrected and best-corrected vision, manifest, and cycloplegic refraction. If irregular astigmatism is present, a hard contact lens over-refraction can be helpful in screening patients for PTK. Individuals demonstrating 4 or more lines of visual acuity improvement are predicted to have greater benefit with corneal smoothing; hence, they are considered excellent candidates for PTK. CS measurements can be helpful in selecting patients with visual complaints related to reduced contrast but good Snellen vision.

Refractive error is an essential component of selection criteria for PTK because PTK can change corneal curvature dramatically, inducing large refractive errors. Patients with preoperative myopia may benefit from induced hyperopia from corneal curvature flattening from a central ablation; however, patients with preoperative hyperopia will have an increase in their refractive error. Conversely, paracentral ablations will induce relative central corneal steepening, leading to increased myopia. Excessive PTK in the paracentral cornea can also induce unwanted astigmatism at the edge of the ablation zone. Given the risk of anisometropia, contact lens status should be documented. Patients should be informed that with induced anisometropia, contact lenses might be necessary for best-corrected vision. If there is documented contact lens intolerance, lamellar or penetrating keratoplasty may be necessary.

The endpoint of PTK treatment is best established with slit lamp examination. The advantage of laser ablation providing submicron precision is fully utilized by frequent intraoperative slit lamp evaluations. This allows for greater control in order to provide a smooth ablation with minimal refractive error change. The goal is to achieve optimal treatment of pathology by removing a minimal amount of tissue while allowing the patient's epithelium to grow and create a smooth tear-air interface for refraction. Most often, what appears to be an undertreatment is adequate and preserves the option for retreatment in the future.

Always Remember…

Hard contact lens over-refraction is helpful in predicting corneal surface irregularity and in screening patients for PTK.

Central corneal ablation can lead to induced hyperopia, and paracentral corneal ablation can lead to induced myopia.

The Golden Rule in PTK: "An undertreatment is better than an overtreatment."

PEARL #28: MASKING AGENTS FOR SMOOTHER ABLATION

Most indications for PTK involve pathological conditions associated with irregular corneal surface. Thus, the goal of PTK is to smooth over the irregular peaks and valleys. The laser produces a flat beam profile that simply applies the laser energy directly to the irregular corneal surface, creating a thinner cornea with the same irregular surface. Therefore, in order to achieve a smooth ablation, the valleys can be protected with a masking agent while the peaks are preferentially ablated. Masking agents with moderate viscosity and high absorbency at the laser wavelength are ideal. A moderately viscous fluid will cover the irregular surface uniformly and will leave a smoother surface after treatment. High-viscosity agents will not uniformly cover an irregular surface, resist leveling with ablation, and cover peaks as well as valleys. Masking agents may also reduce the degree of PTK-induced hyperopia.

The ideal masking agent will depend on the nature of the corneal pathological condition and on the depth and width of the valleys and peaks. Accordingly, the surgeon should have several masking agents of various viscosities available during surgery. Tears Naturale II (Alcon Laboratories, Fort Worth, Tex) has high absorbency and moderate viscosity, resulting in a relatively smooth ablation. Methylcellulose has high absorbency and is available in three different viscosities. Initially, 2.5% methylcellulose can be used for ablations with large peaks and valleys. The high viscosity allows it to stay in the deep valleys during the ablation of the high peaks and serves to protect normal areas of cornea that should not be exposed to the laser. For most ablations, Celluvisc (1% methylcellulose) (Allergan, Irvine, Calif) has the advantage of being moderately viscous and will stay in valleys more uniformly. A thin layer of Celluvisc can be applied with a microsponge so that it flows off the peaks and stays in the valleys. This can be repeated, with constant reassessment of the surface irregularity, during ablation. A final treatment with Cellufresh (0.5% methylcellulose) (Allergan, Irvine, Calif) can be performed for enhancing the smooth ablation.

An ideal masking agent will not only cover valleys while exposing peaks but also ablate at the same rate as the corneal tissue (Figure 6-2). Because none of the commercially available agents meets all the criteria, many studies are investigating collagen-derived corneal masks. Initial reports are promising in that they are able to provide a smooth corneal surface for optimal visual results.

The type of pathology is an important determinant of tissue ablation rates and the amount of laser energy required. It is important to remember that not only do the normal layers of the cornea ablate at different rates, but different pathologic changes also ablate at different rates from each other and from the surrounding normal corneal tissue. For example, amyloid in lattice dystrophy ablates at a different rate than the surrounding normal stroma, and a corneal scar ablates at a different rate than a calcium plaque associated with band keratopathy. Therefore, more masking agent and energy may be required to treat one portion of the treatment zone compared to another to prevent an irregular surface with a poor visual outcome.

Patients with diffuse, smooth, anterior corneal opacities such as Reis-Buckler's, lattice, and other dystrophies are treated with a wide diameter spot size (eg, 5 to 6 mm) and peripheral ablation zone smoothing with movement of the head to reduce refractive change. Epithelium is removed with the laser unless there is an irregular surface. Masking agents can be used if surface irregularities are noted on intraoperative slit lamp examinations. Discrete, elevated lesions such as Salzmann's nodular degeneration and fibrous nodules in keratoconus can be treated directly with a small, spot-size ablation zone. The

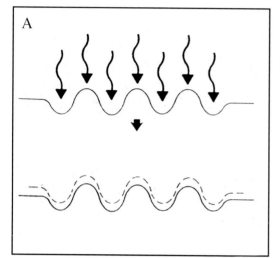
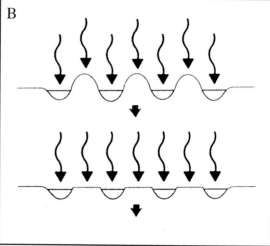

Figure 6-2 (Pearl 28). (A) An irregular surface ablated without fluid will maintain the irregular contour as ablation continues into the deeper stroma. (B) The ideal fluid will have adequate absorption and moderate viscosity to result in ablation of the peaks while masking the valleys. (Reprinted with permission from the American Medical Association. Kornmehl EW, Steinert RF, Puliafito CA. A comparative study of masking fluids for excimer laser phototherapeutic keratectomy. *Arch Ophthalmol.* 1991;109:860-863.)

epithelium over the treatment zone may be removed mechanically; the masking agent is applied to the surrounding normal epithelium preoperatively for the prevention of excessive ablation. Patients with multiple, unevenly distributed lesions are treated with removal of the epithelium and use of masking agents to improve surface smoothness. The masking agents are locally applied to irregular areas followed by varying spot-size ablations.

Always Remember...

> *Masking agents enhance visual outcomes by providing smoother ablations.*

> *Masking agents with different degrees of viscosity can be used in combination for protecting the valleys while ablating the peaks.*

> *Preoperative knowledge of the type of pathology and its ablation properties will aid in planning an effective ablation.*

PEARL #29: PHOTOTHERAPEUTIC KERATECTOMY AND THE RECURRENT EROSION LADDER

Recurrent corneal erosion is a common problem that can occur spontaneously after superficial corneal trauma or secondary to anterior basement membrane dystrophy (Figure 6-3). Typically, the treatment is conservative (eg, lubrication, bandage contact lens), but refractory cases are managed with manual epithelial debridement and anterior stromal puncture. However, patients who do not respond to these treatments or in whom these conventional therapies are contraindicated, including patients with central erosions where anterior stromal puncture may lead to central corneal scarring, may be good candidates for PTK. PTK can be performed between erosion episodes or in the acute phase. Most

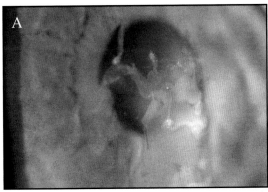
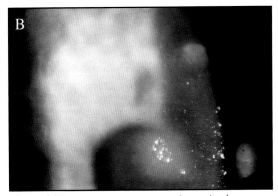

Figure 6-3 (Pearl 29). (A) Map dot fingerprint (MDF) dystrophy and (B) an acute recurrent erosion episode.

studies recommend epithelial debridement prior to laser treatment, especially with acute episodes where irregular epithelium will lead to an irregular ablation. The poorly adherent epithelium overlying the region of the erosion is aggressively debrided with a dry nonfragmenting sponge. An ablation zone large enough to cover the entire debrided area is chosen, with ablation depth ranging from 3 to 6 μm into the Bowman's layer. The hypothesis is that treating the Bowman's layer provides a new bed for the migrating epithelium and allows for improved hemidesmosomal adhesion complexes. When the area of recurrent erosion crosses the visual axis, the ablation zone should be enlarged to end outside the central 4- to 6-mm pupillary axis to prevent any refractive irregularity. The success rate of PTK in refractory cases of recurrent erosions varies from 60% to 90% with follow-up at 24 months. Given the minimal ablation depth, significant refractive changes are not noted.

Always Remember…

PTK with partial ablation of the Bowman's layer provides good long-term results for refractory recurrent corneal erosions.

PTK is preferable compared to stromal punctures in cases of recurrent erosions secondary to anterior basement membrane dystrophy. This will avoid a continuous chase of a diffuse corneal pathology. The opposite is true for traumatic etiologies where the disease is localized.

BIBLIOGRAPHY

Azar DT, Jain S, Stark W. Phototherapeutic keratectomy. In: Azar DT, ed. *Refractive Surgery*. Stanford, Conn: Appleton & Lange; 1997:501-517.

Hersh PS, Burnstein Y, Carr J, Etwaru G, Mayers M. Excimer laser phototherapeutic keratectomy: surgical strategies and clinical outcomes. *Ophthalmology*. 1996;103:1210-1222.

Stark WJ, Gilbert ML, Gottsch JD, Munnerlyn C. Optical pachymetry in the measurement of anterior corneal disease: an evaluative tool for phototherapeutic keratectomy. *Arch Ophthalmol*. 1990;108:12-13.

Thompson V, Durrie DS, Cavanaugh TB. Philosophy and technique for excimer laser phototherapeutic keratectomy. *J Refract Corneal Surg*. 1993;9(suppl):81-90.

Zuckerman SJ, Aquavella JV, Park SB. Analysis of the efficacy and safety of excimer laser PTK in the treatment of corneal disease. *Cornea*. 1996;15:9-14.

CHAPTER 7

THREE
PEARLS IN EXCIMER LASER CORRECTION
AND HYPEROPIA

Nada S. Jabbur, MD; Samir A. Melki, MD, PhD; and Dimitri T. Azar, MD

Refracting and performing refractive surgery in the case of hyperopes is more challenging than in myopes. Specific difficulties may stem from the presence of latent refractive errors, the greater likelihood of regression, the variable response in secondary (refractive surgery-induced) hyperopia, and the increased propensity for decentered ablations.

PEARL #30: LATENT HYPEROPIA, SPASM OF ACCOMMODATION, AND UNDERCORRECTED ASTIGMATISM

Latent hyperopia is the portion of the hyperopic error that is completely corrected by accommodation and is not measurable by manifest refraction. Latent hyperopia can be fully elicited only by adequate cycloplegia. Other methods of refraction, such as fogging techniques and retinoscopy, may indicate the presence of latent hyperopia but are not always adequate in measuring its full magnitude.

Measurement of latent hyperopia is important during the preoperative evaluation because of its relative frequency, particularly in younger patients. The laser treatment should be based on the cycloplegic refraction or "wet" refraction; however, the difference between the cycloplegic refraction and the tolerated manifest refraction, which represents excessive accommodative tone or spasm of accommodation, should not be part of the laser treatment. Failing to detect an excessive accommodative tone may result in overcorrection and possibly a myopic refractive outcome. A large difference between the manifest and the cycloplegic refraction should warrant a postcycloplegic refraction (ie, "dry" refraction on a subsequent day) to verify whether the patient would tolerate the higher dioptric power, which is uncovered by the cycloplegic refraction.

Finally, if an aberrometer is available, one can also take a cluster of measurements not only to check the amount of hyperopia but also the magnitude of astigmatism, which is often underestimated in the manifest and cycloplegic refractions. One can then repeat a postaberrometry refraction and may possibly uncover a more accurate refraction very close in spherical equivalent to the first refraction.

Always Remember...

If the difference between the manifest (push-plus) and cycloplegic measurements is large, a postcycloplegic manifest refraction should be performed to determine whether there is spasm of accommodation and to verify whether the patient is able to tolerate the full cycloplegic prescription.

Fashioning an artificial 3-mm pupil at the phoropter may be useful to minimize distortions originating from the peripheral cornea after pupillary dilation.

Whether the ablation used is conventional or customized, take advantage of an aberrometer refraction to refine the magnitude of hyperopia and astigmatism.

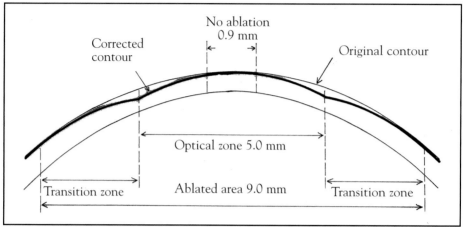

Figure 7-1 (Pearl 31). Diagram of a typical excimer laser hyperopic ablation.

Pearl #31: Hyperopic LASIK: The Importance of Eye Tracking

Irregular and induced astigmatism after hyperopic LASIK seems to occur with higher frequency than following LASIK for myopia. They are associated with loss of BCVA, glare, halos, and lower patient satisfaction. Meticulous centration of the laser ablation and careful realignment of the LASIK flap may minimize these problems.

Surgical procedures performed on the cornea should be centered on the entrance pupil. The entrance pupil is the (virtual) image of the pupil formed by the optical system of the eye. It is located 0.5-mm anterior to and 14% larger than the real pupil is. Decentered laser ablations usually result in loss of BCVA, glare, and visually significant irregular astigmatism. The use of eye tracking technology has revolutionized the treatment of hyperopic errors and minimized the likelihood of poor outcomes associated with decentered hyperopic treatments. This is especially important in hyperopic ablations, which may take 3 times as long to perform as compared to corresponding myopic treatments and have greater potential for fixation loss and uneven stromal bed dehydration. It takes an even longer time if it is a customized ablation with variable spot sizes as it corresponds to a deeper ablation.

A prerequisite for a well-centered ablation in hyperopic LASIK starts with a well-centered corneal flap. A hyperopic ablation is typically 9.0 mm in diameter (Figure 7-1), requiring a larger diameter (>9.0 mm) suction ring. This leaves little room for flap decentration to allow for a full stromal treatment. Corneal curvature is often flat in patients with higher levels of hyperopia, rendering LASIK more challenging due to resulting smaller diameter flaps. Centering the ablation over the pupil should take precedence over avoiding collateral laser damage to the peripheral epithelium or the underside of the reflected flap. Laser ablation beyond the stroma barely diminishes the refractive effect. Ablation of the underside of the flap should be avoided because it can result in an area with double-treatment and irregular astigmatism. Using a flap protector or simply blocking that area by using a large enough instrument in a circular motion to blend the edges of the protected area may minimize the latter (Figure 7-2). Another strategy to avoid the overlapping effect on the flap is to decenter the original suction ring prior to flap creation in the direction of the hinge (Figure 7-3). This may occasionally result in bleeding from the severed limbal vessels (Figure 7-4).

Another problem contributing to corneal irregularity and loss of BCVA after LASIK is inappropriate flap repositioning. This occurs more frequently in hyperopic LASIK than in myopic LASIK because of the increased surface area of the hyperopic flap. Careful and deliberate stroking of the corneal flap with a wet microsponge at the end of the procedure is important for proper realignment.

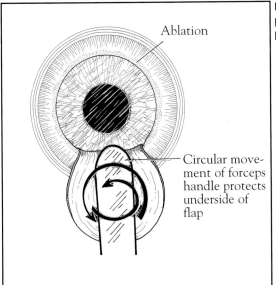

Ablation

Circular movement of forceps handle protects underside of flap

Figure 7-2 (Pearl 31). A forceps handle may be used to protect the underside of the LASIK flap to avoid superposed ablation of stromal tissue.

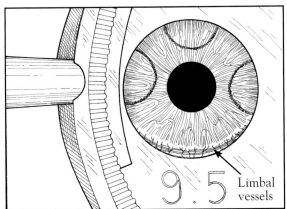

9.5

Limbal vessels

Figure 7-3 (Pearl 31). Superior decentration of the keratome (Hansatome) suction ring has a better chance of exposing a stromal diameter equal to or larger than the laser ablation zone.

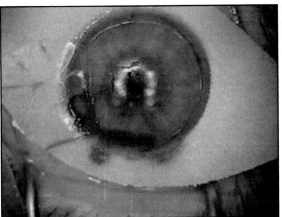

Figure 7-4 (Pearl 31). Creating a larger flap for hyperopic ablations may sever limbal vessels and result in bleeding. This can be controlled with gentle pressure on the cut vessels with a microsponge soaked with naphazoline (eg, Naphcon-A).

Pearl #32: Hyperopic Photorefractive Keratectomy: The Epithelial Challenge

Even though hyperopic LASIK has gradually replaced hyperopic PRK mainly due to better refractive stability in higher corrections, quicker visual rehabilitation, and minimal postoperative discomfort, PRK offers some advantages compared to LASIK. These advantages include corneas with steep preoperative keratometry readings to avoid LASIK flap buttonholes, patients with a history of recurrent corneal erosions, and eyes with a small lid fissure where the suction ring may not fit properly around the cornea.

The challenge with hyperopic PRK is both the removal and the regeneration of the epithelium. One technique to loosen the corneal epithelium is to place a corneal pledget soaked with an anesthetic agent for 90 seconds. Subsequent to that, the use of a blade or the Amoils brush can be helpful to start peeling away the epithelium. The inferior epithelium is often the toughest to remove. It requires the use of a blade or a Paton's spatula. An alternative technique involves exposing the epithelium to 20% alcohol for about 20 seconds followed by epithelial peeling using a microsponge.

The bandage contact lens placed postoperatively should not be removed for at least 4 days even if the central epithelium appears healed. Leaving the contact lens in place for 7 to 10 days will provide adequate time for the epithelial anchoring and may minimize recurrence of the defect.

Always Remember...

Centering the ablation over the pupil takes precedence over avoiding collateral laser damage to the peripheral epithelium or the underside of the reflected LASIK flap.

The epithelium in a hyperopic PRK ablation can be difficult to remove because of the larger and well-adhered peripheral area, especially inferiorly.

The epithelium may be loose even 4 days postoperatively, and premature removal of a bandage contact lens may slow down the healing or enlarge the defect.

Bibliography

Anschutz T. Laser correction of hyperopia and presbyopia. *Int Ophthalmol Clin.* 1994;34:103-137.

Jackson WB, Casson E, Hodge WG, Mintsioulis G, Agapitos PJ. Laser vision correction for low hyperopia: an 18-month assessment of safety and efficacy. *Ophthalmology.* 1998;105:1727-1738.

Jackson WB, Mintsioulis G, Agapitos PJ, Casson EJ. Excimer laser photorefractive keratectomy for low hyperopia: safety and efficacy. *J Cataract Refract Surg.* 1997;23:480-487.

Primack JD, Azar DT. Refractive surgery for hyperopia. *Int Ophthalmol Clin.* 2000;40(3):151-163.

Uozato H, Guyton DL. Centering corneal surgical procedures. *Am J Ophthalmol.* 1987;103(3[Pt 1]):264-275.

CHAPTER 8

Two Irregular Astigmatism Pearls

Ramon C. Ghanem, MD; Faisal Al-Tobaigy, MD; Elena Albè, MD; and Dimitri T. Azar, MD

PEARL #33: SECONDARY HYPEROPIA AND IRREGULAR ASTIGMATISM AFTER RADIAL KERATOTOMY AND DECENTERED ABLATION

Before the advent of excimer laser refractive surgery, RK was widely used to correct myopia in United States and worldwide. In RK, partial-thickness radial incisions are made in the paracentral and peripheral cornea using a diamond-bladed micrometer knife. These incisions cause a weakening of the peripheral cornea with consequent flexing and a compensatory flattening of the central cornea. However, with time, biomechanical weakening of the mid-peripheral cornea seems to develop, leading to progressive peripheral steepening and central flattening, resulting in secondary progressive hyperopia frequently associated with irregular astigmatism. Results from the Prospective Evaluation of Radial Keratotomy Study (PERK Study) showed that, between 6 months and 10 years after treatment, 43% of eyes had a hyperopic shift of 1.00 D or more with no tendency towards stability.

Noncustomized photoablative techniques have been proposed for the treatment of this condition. Favorable results were observed with intrastromal ablation (ie, LASIK) and with PRK. However, many complications were reported with LASIK, namely opening the RK incisions during the flap lift, epithelial ingrowth in the interface, and DLK. Another important concern when performing LASIK after RK is the possible augmentation of the inherent corneal instability present in post-RK eyes. With PRK, however, the main complication is the risk of postoperative haze with loss of BCVA and CS.

To overcome these obstacles, we use topography supported PRK (TOSCA [Topography Supported Customized Ablation] Asclepion-Meditec AG, Jena, Germany) with adjunctive MMC 0.02% intraoperatively (Figures 8-1 and 8-2). The surgical technique consists of chemical epithelium debridement with alcohol 20% for 30 seconds followed by laser ablation (Meditec MEL-70 G-scan flying-spot with TOSCA). After photoablation, a sterile 3-mm circular cellulose sponge soaked in MMC 0.02% is applied to the central corneal surface for 20 seconds followed by irrigation with 20 ml of balanced salt solution. A bandage soft contact lens is then applied for 4 days. Steroid and antibiotic eye drops are used every 2 hours and tapered over 2 months.

The use of topography-guided surface ablation in these cases avoids biomechanical corneal weakening caused by the microkeratome cut through the Bowman's layer and superficial stroma and has the potential to treat irregular corneas with fairly good results. In eyes that have had RK and have shown inherent corneal instability with a progressive shift in refraction due to peripheral corneal weakening, performing a corrective procedure such as LASIK may augment the instability. The long-term effect of weakening the cornea is not known, but it could initiate another shift in refraction or accelerate it. Wavefront-guided ablation is also an alternative to topography-guided ablation since most aberrations of the optical system are localized in the cornea in these patients but data acquisition is usually not reproducible.

Haze is an important complication following surface ablation in eyes with previous RK. The adjunctive use of MMC intraoperatively can significantly decrease the incidence of postoperative central cornea haze. We do not recommend the use of MMC in the whole photoablation area or in the region of the RK incisions. The preceding debridement of the epithelium may induce a gaping of the RK wounds.

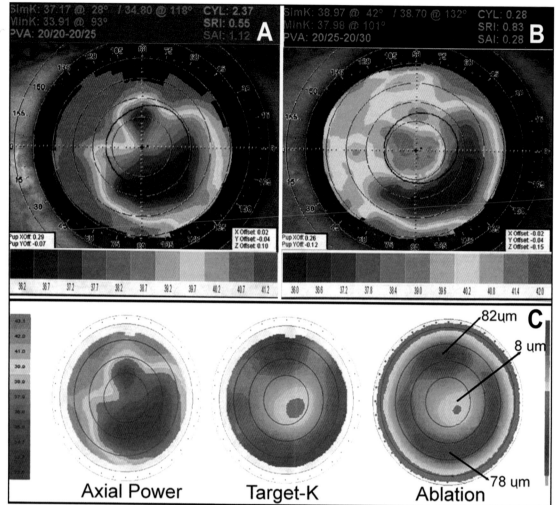

Figure 8-1 (Pearl 33). Secondary hyperopia and irregular astigmatism after RK treated with topographic-guided ablation and adjunctive MMC 0.02% intraoperatively. A 47-year-old male underwent an uncomplicated bilateral RK procedure in 1990. His preoperative refractive error was –1.25 –1.50 x 175 degrees (20/20) and –1.75 –1.50 x 10 degrees (20/20) OD and OS, respectively. In April 2003, 13 years after the RK procedure, the patient was evaluated for complaints of decreased near and distance vision. At that time, uncorrected VA was 20/25 and 20/100, and his refraction was +1.00 –0.75 x 90 degrees (20/20) and +5.00 –1.75 x 95 degrees (20/25) OD and OS, respectively. The patient underwent hyperopic PRK with TOSCA in the left eye as described previously. (A, B) The pre- and postoperative topographies. (C) TOSCA ablation profile.

The penetration of MMC in these incisions may cause a delay in re-epithelization and may avoid the upgrowth of fibrosis in this area, which may be biomechanically disadvantageous.

This technique has been shown to be useful for correcting RK-induced hyperopia with or without irregular astigmatism. It may also be used to treat undercorrected RK patients, since haze is a major concern when treating these patients.

How to Treat Irregular Astigmatism After Decentered Laser Ablation

Irregular astigmatism after excimer laser surgery is usually associated with other complications such as flap folds and striae, DLK, epithelial ingrowth, and decentered ablations. The incidence of decentered ablation has decreased significantly since the advent of reliable eye-tracking systems, but it still can occur if careful attention is not paid to patient fixation or if the ablation is centered on the pupil, but

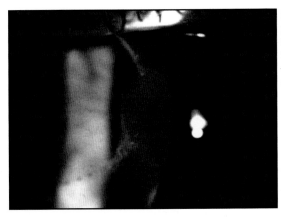

Figure 8-2 (Pearl 33). Moderate haze in the corneal periphery in the area of the incisions 3 months after treatment in the same patient as Figure 8-1. At 12 months, uncorrected VA was 20/40, and the refraction was –1.25 –0.50 x 10 degrees (20/20). Trace haze could still be observed in the corneal periphery.

the visual axis of the eye is largely off center in relation to the pupil (large angle kappa). Clinically significant decentered ablation (usually ≥1.0 mm) can create disturbing visual symptoms; the induced multifocallity on the optical zone can cause monocular diplopia, reduction of BCVA and CS, shadows, and glare, which may increase at night, causing driving difficulties. Possible techniques to treat decentered ablations include masking techniques to expand the ablation zone, combined decentered myopic and hyperopic ablations, transepithelial ablation opposite to the decentered ablation, and customized ablations. Both wavefront-guided ablation and topographic-linked ablation are good options for these patients. However, as mentioned before, reliable wavefront data cannot be acquired in most patients with irregular corneas. Our choice in these cases is also topographic-linked ablation using TOSCA (Figure 8-3), but other topographic-linked laser systems can be used as well.

Always Remember…

Avoid Mitomycin application beyond the central 3 mm in corneas with previous RK incisions.

PEARL #34: TREATMENT OF KERATECTASIA IN KERATOCONUS FOLLOWING LASIK

Keratectasia is a major sight-threatening complication following refractive surgery. Keratectasia results from changes in corneal biomechanical stability induced by laser ablation especially after LASIK. The LASIK flap does not contribute to the corneal biomechanical stability after LASIK surgery, leaving a weaker area in the cornea, rendering it more vulnerable to pressure distortion effect compared to other parts of the ocular wall, and leading to a forward shift of the posterior surface of the cornea. Lowering IOP may help in stabilizing keratectasia.

One of the most common causes of keratectasia following refractive surgery is undiagnosed preoperative forme fruste keratoconus. Other causes include high ablation depth and low residual bed thickness.

Preoperative evaluation of refractive surgery candidates is the mainstay for successful refractive surgery results. Two main issues are of particular importance: careful analysis of topographic data and precise calculation of surgical parameters. Curvature topographic maps as well as elevation maps are important to exclude any kind of corneal irregularities and corneal ectasia. Central corneal pachymetry, ablation zone, ablation depth, flap thickness, and remaining residual stromal bed are the most important parameters to be known preoperatively. Flap thickness may differ from the desired thickness by 30 µm or more. For that reason, intraoperative pachymetry of the remaining bed before the ablation is helpful to calculate the residual bed thickness. The remaining stromal bed should be not less than 250 µm. If the corneal pachymetry is less than 500 µm, surface ablation may be a better option. For patients with more than 10 D of myopia, corneal refractive procedures may be deferred and other refractive options such as phakic IOL implantation can be considered.

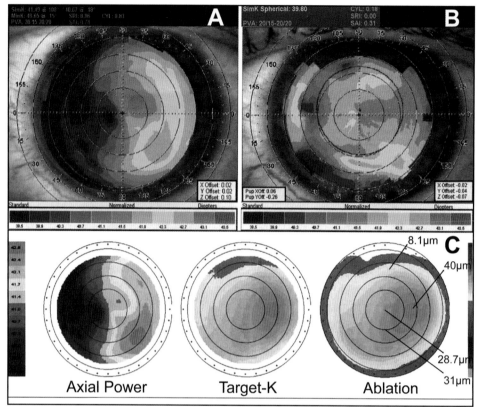

Figure 8-3 (Pearl 33). Irregular astigmatism after decentered LASIK treated with topographic-guided ablation. A 35-year-old male underwent a bilateral myopic LASIK procedure in 1997. The patient was evaluated in 2004 for complaints of reduction of BCVA, night glare, and ghost images in both eyes. On examination, BCVA was 20/40 in both eyes, and his refraction was –2.00 – 1.25 x 65 degrees and –1.00 –0.50 x 40 degrees, OD and OS, respectively. (A, B) Corneal topography revealed severe decentration in both eyes. The patient underwent a bilateral nonsimultaneous TOSCA intrastromal ablation after the flap was lifted. (C, D) TOSCA ablation profile. Arrows indicate the amount of tissue removed in specific areas of the cornea. (E, F) One year postoperative topography. At that time, the patient reported resolution of the disturbing visual symptoms. Uncorrected VA was 20/30 and 20/25, and the refraction was –0.50 x 80 degrees (20/25) and plano, OD and OS, respectively.

A clinical diagnosis of keratectasia can be suspected when a patient develops unstable vision associated with irregular astigmatism. It usually occurs 6 to 18 months after LASIK surgery, but it may occur at any time.

The treatment options for postoperative keratectasia are similar to the treatment of primary keratoconus. Rigid gas permeable contact lens is the best option and can provide good visual rehabilitation if the patient can tolerate it. Some data has shown an improvement of visual acuity and stabilization of vision in patients with keratectasia following complicated excimer laser photo ablation using flap sutures. It is not recommended to treat keratectasia with irregular astigmatism by laser custom ablation, which may lead to further thinning and worsening of the condition.

Intrastromal corneal rings are a good option for patients with iatrogenic keratectasia and keratoconus who are contact lens intolerant with a clear visual axis. It can delay the need for corneal transplants or eliminate it. It is a good surgical option to consider because it has lower rates of complications compared to deep anterior lamellar keratoplasty (DALK) or penetrating keratoplasty. Femtosecond laser has made the insertion of the corneal rings even easier with exact planned depth. There are two kinds of stromal

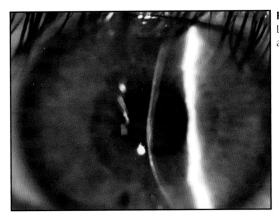

Figure 8-4 (Pearl 34). Iatrogenic keratectasia after myopic LASIK. Note inferior corneal steepening and thinning characteristics of advanced keratectasia.

segments: the INTACS and Ferrara rings. INTACS are inserted through a 1.8-mm corneal incision and have a 7-mm optical zone. Ferrara rings have a triangular cross-section and provide an optical zone of 5.0 mm. Most of the time, two segments are implanted facing each other with different thicknesses to balance the irregular astigmatism according to the manufacturer nomogram, and in some situations, one segment can be used. Although the predictability of the procedure is not high, the UCVA becomes significantly better than preoperatively for most patients. The corneal segments act by reshaping the cornea and make the steep cornea flatter, allowing for contact lens wear. Postoperative topical steroids, antibiotics, and tears should be used for 2 weeks. It is exchangeable and removable without affecting the central cornea. Unsatisfied patients can still undergo other surgical options such as DALK or penetrating keratoplasty.

Always Remember...

It may be worth considering intracorneal rings prior to more invasive procedures in treating corneal ectasia.

BIBLIOGRAPHY

Alessio G, Boscia F, La Tegola MG, et al. Topography-driven photorefractive keratectomy: results of corneal interactive programmed topographic ablation software. *Ophthalmology.* 2000;107(8):1578-1587.

Alio JL, Artola A, Rodriguez-Mier FA. Selective zonal ablations with excimer laser for correction of irregular astigmatism induced by refractive surgery. *Ophthalmology.* 2000;107(4):662-673.

Alio JL, Belda JI, Osman AA, et al. Topography-guided laser in situ keratomileusis (TOPOLINK) to correct irregular astigmatism after previous refractive surgery. *J Refract Surg.* 2003;19(5):516-527.

Alkara N, Genth U, Seiler T. Diametral ablation—a technique to manage decentered photorefractive keratectomy for myopia. *J Refract Surg.* 1999;15(4):436-440.

Anwar M, Teichmann KD. Big-bubble technique to bare Descemet's membrane in anterior lamellar keratoplasty. *J Cataract Refract Surg.* 2002;28(3):398-403.

Azar DT, Tuli S, Benson RA, et al. Photorefractive keratectomy for residual myopia after radial keratotomy. PRK After RK Study Group. *J Cataract Refract Surg.* 1998;24(3):303-311.

Colin J, Velou S. Current surgical options for keratoconus. *J Cataract Refract Surg.* 2003;29(2):379-386.

Francesconi CM, Nose RA, Nose W. Hyperopic laser-assisted in situ keratomileusis for radial keratotomy induced hyperopia. *Ophthalmology.* 2002;109(3):602-605.

Guell JL, Velasco F. Topographically guided ablations for the correction of irregular astigmatism after corneal surgery. *Int Ophthalmol Clin.* 2003;43(3):111-128.

Guirao A. Theoretical elastic response of the cornea to refractive surgery: risk factors for keratectasia. *J Refract Surg.* 2005;21(2):176-185.

Jaycock PD, Lobo L, Ibrahim J, Tyrer J, Marshall J. Interferometric technique to measure biomechanical changes in the cornea induced by refractive surgery. *J Cataract Refract Surg.* 2005;31(1):175-184.

Joyal H, Gregoire J, Faucher A. Photorefractive keratectomy to correct hyperopic shift after radial keratotomy. *J Cataract Refract Surg.* 2003;29:1502–1506.

Knorz MC, Jendritza B. Topographically-guided laser in situ keratomileusis to treat corneal irregularities. *Ophthalmology.* 2000;107(6):1138-1143.

Kymionis GD, Panagopoulou SI, Aslanides IM, et al. Topographically supported customized ablation for the management of decentered laser in situ keratomileusis. *Am J Ophthalmol.* 2004;137(5):806-811.

Lafond G, Bonnet S, Solomon L. Treatment of previous decentered excimer laser ablation with combined myopic and hyperopic ablations. *J Refract Surg.* 2004;20(2):139-148.

Leaming DV. Practice styles and preferences of ASCRS members—1990 survey. *J Cataract Refract Surg.* 1991;17(4):495-502.

Lin DY, Manche EE. Custom-contoured ablation pattern method for the treatment of decentered laser ablations. *J Cataract Refract Surg.* 2004;30(8):1675-1684.

Lipshitz I, Man O, Shemesh G, et al. Laser in situ keratomileusis to correct hyperopic shift after radial keratotomy. *J Cataract Refract Surg.* 2001;27(2):273-276.

Majmudar PA, Forstot SL, Dennis RF, et al. Topical Mitomycin-C for subepithelial fibrosis after refractive corneal surgery. *Ophthalmology.* 2000;107(1):89-94.

Maloney RK, Chan WK, Steinert R, et al. A multicenter trial of photorefractive keratectomy for residual myopia after previous ocular surgery. Summit Therapeutic Refractive Study Group. *Ophthalmology.* 1995;102(7):1042-1052; discussion 1052-1053.

Maloney RK, Chan WK, Steinert R, et al. A multicenter trial of photorefractive keratectomy for residual myopia after previous ocular surgery. Summit Therapeutic Refractive Study Group. *Ophthalmology.* 1995;102(7):1042-52; discussion 1052-1053.

Meza J, Perez-Santonja JJ, Moreno E, et al. Photorefractive keratectomy after radial keratotomy. *J Cataract Refract Surg.* 1994;20(5):485-489.

Miyata K, Tokunaga T, Nakahara M, et al. Residual bed thickness and corneal forward shift after laser in situ keratomileusis. *J Cataract Refract Surg.* 2004;30(5):1067-1072.

Morris E, Kirwan JF, Sujatha S, Rostron CK. Corneal endothelial specular microscopy following deep lamellar keratoplasty with lyophilized tissue. *Eye.* 1998;12(4):619-622.

Seo KY, Lee JH, Kim MJ, et al. Effect of suturing on latrogenic keratectasia after laser in situ keratomileusis. *J Refract Surg.* 2004;20(1):40-45.

Silbiger JS, Cohen EJ, Laibson PR. The rate of visual recovery after penetrating keratoplasty for keratoconus. *CLAO J.* 1996;22(4):266-269.

Sugita J, Kondo J. Deep lamellar keratoplasty with complete removal of pathological stroma for vision improvement. *Br J Ophthalmol.* 1997;81(3):184-188.

Toshino A, Uno T, Ohashi Y, Maeda N, Oshika T. Transient keratectasia caused by intraocular pressure elevation after laser in situ keratomileusis. *J Cataract Refract Surg.* 2005;31(1):202-204.

Venter JA. Photorefractive keratectomy for hyperopia after radial keratotomy. *J Refract Surg.* 1997;13(5 Suppl):S456.

Waring GO 3rd, Lynn MJ, McDonnell PJ. Results of the prospective evaluation of radial keratotomy (PERK) study 10 years after surgery. *Arch Ophthalmol.* 1994;112(10):1298-1308.

CHAPTER 9

FOUR PEARLS ON PRESBYOPIC CORRECTION

Elena Albé, MD; Faisal Al-Tobaigy, MD; Ramon C. Ghanem, MD;
Samir A. Melki, MD, PhD; and Dimitri T. Azar, MD

PEARL #35: MONOVISION REFRACTIVE SURGERY

Monovision is a method of presbyopic correction whereby one eye is corrected for distance vision and the other eye for near vision. Conventional monovision refers to correction of the dominant eye for distance and the nondominant eye for near. Crossed monovision refers to correction of the dominant eye for near and the nondominant eye for distance. The choice of which eye is corrected for distance may depends on patients' needs and occupation. Several theories were proposed for selection of the corrected distance eye: (1) correcting the dominant eye to maximize visual performance and activities such as driving, (2) correcting the dominant eye to produce smaller esophoric shift at distance, (3) correcting the left eye for increased driving safety, and (4) correcting the less myopic eye. The dominant eye generally is identified by use of sighting dominance tests. One of the more common tests is the hole test, whereby the patient, using both eyes simultaneously, lines up an object through a hole, usually formed by the patient's hands. As the patient constricts the size of the hole, the eye that continues to be aligned with the object and the hole is considered to be the dominant eye.

Currently, monovision may be achieved through contact lens use, IOLs, conductive keratoplasty (CK), or refractive techniques such as LASIK, PRK, LASEK or Epi-LASIK. In mild myopic patients, monovision may also be achieved by correcting only one eye for distance, leaving the other eye untreated. The amount of under correction in myopic monovision patients varies according to the age of the patient, ranging from 1.25 D to 2.5 D.

The goal of monovision is to give comfortable unaided functional vision. Nevertheless, spectacle correction may be needed for certain tasks in which binocular distance or near vision is required, like in night driving or prolonged near tasks. The monovision patient should be able to see clearly at all distances. Inherent to the monovision concept is the fact that at any given distance, the image in one eye will be blurred and the image in the other eye in focus. Ideally, at any given distance, a patient should be able to suppress the blurred image from one eye so that it does not interfere with the image from the other eye (interocular blur suppression). Blur suppression aids distance binocular vision, so that only a slight reduction in distance acuity occurs.

Patients' acceptance after monovision refractive surgery has been reported to range between 72% and 92.5%. Careful patient selection and counseling is very important in monovision refractive surgery. All patients who opt for monovision must be informed of the adverse effect monovision may have on some visual function parameters. Specifically, they need to be informed of the risk of reduced binocular visual acuity, stereoacuity, and CS. In addition, they need to be made aware of the risk of glare and distance and near ghosting as a result of incomplete blur suppression. Blur suppression appears to be particularly problematic under night driving conditions because interocular blur suppression becomes less effective under dim illumination conditions. Therefore, patients must be advised of the need to wear distance glasses when driving. Poor candidates for monovision are patients who exhibit minimal intraocular suppression of blur, patients with large esophoric shifts with monovision, and patients with a significant reduction in stereoacuity with monocular correction.

Always Remember...

Crossed monovision refers to relying on the nondominant eye for distance vision and may be well tolerated.

PEARL #36: CONDUCTIVE KERATOPLASTY, MONOVISION, AND BLENDED VISION

Conductive Keratoplasty: Light Touch Technique

CK is a nonablative, nonlamellar technique in which low radiofrequency energy (350 kHz) is applied with a probe tip to the peripheral corneal stroma. During each application, RF energy is delivered into the cornea for 0.6 seconds at an energy level of 0.6 watts. The inherent electrical impedance of the corneal stroma results in heating of the tissue to approximately 65°C, the optimal temperature for collagen shrinkage. A full circle of CK spots applied to the corneal midperiphery causes peripheral flattening and central steepening, inducing a myopic shift to the eye. The effect of CK is determined by the number of spots (8, 16, or 24) and the optical zone of the treatment (6 mm, 7 mm, and/or 8 mm). The treatment pattern and number of spots is based on the current "light-touch technique" nomogram. According to this technique, some pressure is applied when inserting the Keratoplast tip (Refractec, Irvine, Calif) into the stroma, but after the tip is inserted, the pressure is released and the foot pedal is depressed to administer the energy. With the previous technique, some pressure had to be applied to the cornea during treatment ("firm pressure" technique). Late undercorrection was common, and uneven pressure in different spots could result in induced astigmatism. After the introduction of the new technique, the CK nomogram was changed because greater amounts of correction could be achieved with the application of fewer spots. Also, for the same amount of correction, a larger optical zone can be used, sparing the 6 mm (central) zone when possible. For example, a +1.75 hyperopic eye would need 24 spots divided in the 6-, 7-, and 8-mm optical zone with the previous technique. With the light-touch technique, for the same correction, only 8 spots in the 7-mm optical zone must be applied.

NearVision CK (Refractec) is indicated for the temporary improvement of near vision in emmetropic presbyopes (those who require only reading glasses) and hyperopic presbyopes (those who require reading and distance glasses). The procedure is typically performed on just one eye, improving near vision without substantially compromising the patient's binocular distance vision. Candidates for CK should have correctable distance visual acuity to at least 20/40 in both eyes and near visual acuity correctable to at least J3 in the nondominant eye. They should be 40 years of age or older and require a presbyopic add of +1.00 to +2.00 D.

Contraindications include peripheral pachymetry reading less than 560 μm (measured at the 6-mm optical zone) central corneal scarring, pregnant, lactating, or nursing women.

At the end of the procedure, the patient may experience some foreign body sensation, tearing, dry eye, and fluctuation in vision for a few weeks after the procedure. A case of partially brown-colored corneal iron ring located between the CK-treated spots has been described and related to the alterations in tear film stability caused by CK-induced changes in corneal curvature. CK results may not be permanent for a natural presbyopic progression, and as they age, patients may again require reading glasses. CK retreatments may be performed, but results of retreatments have not been rigorously assessed to date.

In an attempt to look at the clinical safety and effectiveness of CK for the treatment of presbyopia, a Phase III multicenter clinical trial was performed with the Refractec Viewpoint Conductive Keratoplasty system (Refractec Inc, Irvine, Calif) studying 150 consecutive subjects. As in clinical use today, the treatment plan was designed to correct the nondominant eye for near vision. Thus, patients without distance vision problems usually require only one eye to be treated. Those with hyperopia in the other eye may require bilateral treatment.

No clinically or statistically significant changes in endothelial cell count from preoperative levels have been observed after CK. The application of CK after previous refractive procedures is under investigation. One case of corneal and iris perforation with anterior capsule opacification has been reported by

Kymionis et al, after CK on a patient with a previous arcuate keratotomy and LASIK. One case report by Klein et al suggested that LASIK can be safely performed after CK. In their last paper, Kymionis et al reported that the treatment of hyperopia with LASIK in an eye with refractive regression following previous CK resulted in a predicted refractive outcome with no complications and improvement in visual acuity at 6 months follow-up. A larger case series is necessary to confirm these findings and to better ascertain flap-related topographic and refractive effects of previous CK.

Always Remember …

Light touch CK allows the same level of correction with fewer treatment spots.

The result of CK is not different from monovision. Consider a preoperative contact lens trial when appropriate.

PEARL #37: SCLERAL SURGERY FOR PRESBYOPIA

Two kinds of scleral surgery for presbyopia are currently performed: scleral expansion band (SEB) and anterior ciliary sclerotomy (ACS). Both techniques aim to increase the scleral diameter surgically. The mechanism by which these surgeries exert their effect is controversial, with disagreement about the accommodative process. In 1855, Helmotz proposed that accommodation occurs because of the elastic property of the lens that allows it to be more convex when the zonular tension is relieved during ciliary muscle contraction.

Another theory described by Tshering proposed that zonular tension rather than relaxation may be the mechanism of accommodation. Schachar modified this theory and suggested that accommodation occurs because of the elastic property of the lens that allows it to be more convex when the zonulat tension is increased during ciliary muscle contraction. He also proposed that the distance between the lens capsule equator and the ciliary body decreases with age. This led him to suggest that by expanding the scleral wall around the lens equator, the ciliary body working distance would also be increased, allowing more pulling effect on the equatorial zonules.

SEB involves placing four polymethylmethacrylate (PMMA) segments into partial-thickness scleral pockets in each of the four oblique quadrants of the eye posterior to the limbus in order to expand the sclera over the ciliary muscle. For proper scleral expansion, the SEB should be placed tightly in a scleral pocket 50% or more of the scleral depth, 4 mm long, and 1.5 mm wide. This might not be reproducible manually every time, and if not, it may lead to extrusion, rotation, or exert no scleral expansion at all. An electromechanical machine, Presbydrive (Presby Corp, Dallas, Tex), is available to make ideal scleral pockets. When the automated pockets are used, these segments can produce 300 μm of radial scleral expansion along the plane of the crystalline lens equator. This expansion is claimed to result in approximately 7 D of accommodative amplitude.

Although some data showed improvement in near vision clinically after SEB, other reports showed that improved near vision is not universal nor long lasting, and it may be related to multifocality rather than through accommodation. Another report measured the accommodation subjectively and objectively in a satisfied bilateral SEB patient. They found no increase in accommodative amplitude above normal age matched controls.

The available clinical data regarding SEB effectiveness, patients' satisfaction, and safety profile is not encouraging for it to be considered as treatment for presbyopia. It can cause mild or florid anterior segment ischemia, transient IOP elevation, tear film disturbance, and conjunctival scarring. The segments can erode the scleral tissue, overlying it, or compromise the glaucoma filtration or retinal detachment surgeries should the need arise later in life.

ACS is a procedure in which radial scleral cuts are made with a diamond knife or laser ablation over the ciliary body to allow the sclera to expand. In theory, this may enhance the space between the crystalline lens and the ciliary body. The procedure was first described by Thornton and modified by Fukasaku when he added a silicone implant into the scleral incision to enhance its effect and stabilize the wound for longer time.

ACS involves eight equally spaced radial incisions of the sclera overlying the ciliary body, two in each oblique quadrant. Limbal peritomies overlying the oblique quadrants avoid excessive conjunctival bleeding and, more importantly, allow accurate measurement of the length and the depth of the incisions. Ultrasonic biomicroscopy (UBM) has been introduced to accurately measure the depth of the incision, the scleral thickness (670 µm), and the setting for blade depth prior to incision of the sclera. A diamond knife or infrared laser can be used to perform scleral incisions that are 95% to 100% of its thickness. The incision length is 3.0 mm and starts 1 mm posterior to the surgical limbus to adequately include the sclera overlying the ciliary body and posterior chamber without unnecessarily incising sclera overlying uvea and retina.

Fakusaku and Marron reported a good initial postoperative effect from this procedure with a mean increase in accommodative amplitude of 2.2 D. The effect of the procedure was gradually decreased, with only 0.8 D of gain in accommodative amplitude remaining at 1 year postoperative. They attributed the fading effect of the procedure to scleral wound healing, which led them to introduce silicon plugs in the incisions to prevent scleral healing. These plugs reduced this regression, with a mean accommodative amplitude gain of 1.5 D at 12 months. Hamilton and coauthors found that ACS has no effect in restoring accommodation.

Potential intraoperative and postoperative complications may occur in these kind of full-thickness ocular wall incisions. Anterior segment perforation, aqueous leak, endophthalmitis, mild or florid anterior segment ischemia with anterior chamber inflammation, iris atrophy, and akinesis are the most serious complications. Scleral incisions may also weaken ocular wall integrity, making it more vulnerable to rupture after blunt trauma compared to normal eyes.

Always Remember…

Scleral surgery for presbyopia is still controversial and is awaiting FDA approval.

PEARL #38: ACCOMMODATING AND MULTIFOCAL INTRAOCULAR LENSES

The ultimate goal of cataract surgery is to replace the cataractous crystalline lens with an IOL that simulates the original function of the crystalline lens and provides the patient with a full range of functional vision for distance and near. Currently, this problem can be addressed by implanting an accommodating or a multifocal IOL. The advantages of astigmatically neutral clear corneal incisions and precise biometry as well as IOL power calculations have allowed for increased utilization of these technologies in both cataract and refractive lens exchange surgery.

Accommodating Intraocular Lenses

The accommodating IOLs are aimed at compensating for the loss of lens accommodation after cataract surgery. However, following cataract surgery, some accommodative functions of the ciliary muscle are retained and pseudoaccommodation would be due to one or a combination of the following: multifocality, monovision, a small pupil resulting in increased depth of focus, and ocular aberrations (by slight against-the-rule astigmatism and spherical aberration).

It has been demonstrated that the ciliary muscle, upon accommodation constriction, undergoes a redistribution of its mass with encroachment into the vitreous cavity. This could provide vitreous pressure against the posterior lens surface, possibly inducing forward movement of an IOL.

Two different IOLs designs concepts have demonstrated accommodative ability:
1. Single optic and flexible haptic support:
    a. Eyeonics AT-45 CrystaLens (Eyeonics Inc, Aliso Viejo, Calif).
    b. 1CU HumanOptics (Human Optics AG, Erlangen, Germany).
2. Dual optical system: Synchrony IOL (Visiogen Inc, Irvine, Calif).

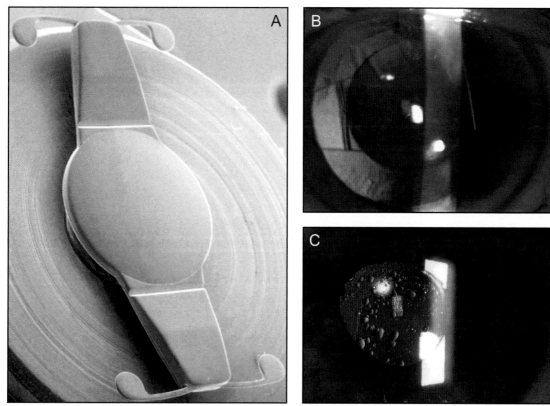

Figure 9-1 (Pearl 38). (A, B) Scanning electron microscopy of Crystalens, which has 4.5 mm silicone optic and an 11.5 mm oval diameter. Adjacent to the optic are grooved plate haptics with ends made of polyamide. (C) One disadvantage of the Crystalens is the silicone makeup that may lead to silicone oil adherence in vitreoretinal surgery. (Courtesy of Samir A. Melki, MD, PhD.)

Eyeonics AT-45 Crystalens

The AT-45 Crystalens accommodating IOL was designed by Stuart Cumming, MD. The theoretical mechanism of action of this lens is based on the concept of accommodation, resulting in a rearrangement of the volume of the ciliary body, which in turn results in rising pressure within the vitreous body. This should move the IOL optic forward along the optical axis, resulting in an IOL with more refractive power.

The Crystalens (Figure 9-1) has a hinged design that might permit forward movement of the optic because of pressure changes in the vitreous cavity.

The review of the outcomes showed that the lens centration has been excellent; there have been few dislocations, and the ability of the patients to see at near and intermediate through their distance correction has been variable but observed consistently in all patients, resulting in excellent patient satisfaction. YAG capsulotomies have been reported to have no effect on the ability of these patients to see at near. Despite the small optic size (4.5 mm), the FDA clinical trial showed that only about 5% of the patients implanted with the Crystalens will have severe nigh-time glare/flare, difficulty driving at night, and/or halos. This is probably due to three factors: the deep placement of the optic within the eye, the excellent centration, and the nonreflective nature of the third-generation silicone material BioSil (BioSil Ltd, Isle of Man, British Isles).

A potential complication with this lens is capsular fibrosis, which could result in anterior movement of the IOL, causing a shift in the refraction to –2.5 D of myopia. Conversely, a decrease in the diameter of the capsular bag could result in posterior lens movement and subsequent hyperopia.

Figure 9-2 (Pearl 38). Humanoptics Akkommodative 1CU IOL consists of hydrophilic acrylate and has an optical diameter of 5.5 mm and an overall diameter of 9.8 mm (scanning electron microscopy).

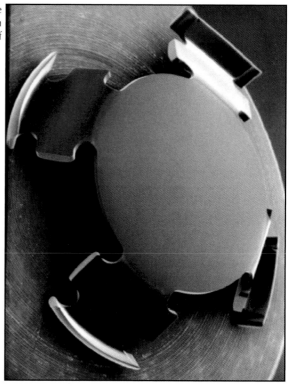

HumanOptics Accommodative 1CU Intraocular Lens

Khalil Hanna designed the HumanOptics accommodating IOL basing his studies on Helmholtz's theory. According to Helmholtz, accommodation occurs when the ciliary muscle contracts, resulting in relaxation of the zonular attachments to the natural crystalline lens. With the relaxation of the zonules, the lens assumes a more spherical shape, leading to an increase in the dioptric power of the retinal plane. When accommodation ceases, relaxation of the ciliary muscle results in an increase in zonular tension. This flattens the shape of the lens, with a subsequent reduction in its dioptric power. This brings distant objects into focus on the retinal plane.

The 1CU (Figure 9-2) has modified haptics that bend in the bag as the lens capsule contracts, which are supposed to cause anterior displacement of the lens optic. The relaxation of the zonular fibers with contraction of the ciliary body leads to relaxation of the capsular bag and forward movement of the IOL at the hinges of the four haptics.

1CU IOL eyes performed better than monofocal IOLs in both distance corrected near visual acuity and subjective near point vision. However, a study by Claoue et al that compared the 1CU IOL with a multifocal IOL found that a greater proportion of Array IOL recipients than 1CU HumanOptics IOL recipients achieved functional near visual acuity.

Dual Optic System Intraocular Lens

Synchrony is a single piece, silicone, dual-optic accommodating IOL for placement inside the capsular bag (Figure 9-3). It is made up of two lenses kept apart by haptics with springlike action. The anterior optic is 5.5 mm large and has a 30 to 35 D optical power; the posterior optic is 6 mm large and a negative power varying depending on ocular axial length. The overall length of the IOL is 9.5 mm, its width is 9.8 mm, and its thickness is 2.2 mm when it is compressed. During the nonaccommodative phase, the taut zonules keep the antero-posterior distance close and the energy in the spring mechanism suppressed. When the ciliary muscle contracts, the zonular fibers relax and the spring releases its energy, driving

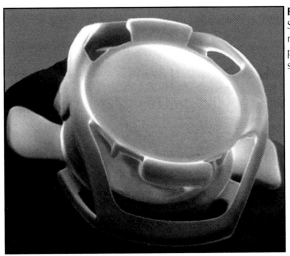

Figure 9-3 (Pearl 38). The single-piece silicone Synchrony IOL features a 5.5-mm high-powered anterior convex optic connected to a 6.0-mm negative power concave posterior optic by haptics that have a springlike action (scanning electron microscopy).

the two lenses apart and, thereby, increasing the antero-posterior distance leading to an accommodative effect. Werner et al showed that the Synchrony accommodating IOL, when compared to a conventional IOL group in rabbit eyes, caused less fibrosis, ACO, and PCO. Although there was a greater incidence of anterior chamber IOL dislocation and pupillary block in the accommodating IOL group versus the control group, possible explanations to this phenomenon may be the relative discrepancy between the IOL size and the relatively small tested animal eyes.

The Synchrony IOL has been reported to have accommodative amplitude of 2.5 D based on a defocus curve. The Synchrony IOL is still in the experimental phase at the time of this publication.

Multifocal Intraocular Lenses

Diffractive multifocal IOLs were the first to gain some diffusion in clinical practice and the first to be evaluated clinically, but they showed significant optical deficiencies that discouraged many ophthalmologists from using them. Bifocal refractive IOLs, with different optical zones devoted to distance and near vision, appeared at the same time. In an attempt to avoid the problems of the first generation multifocal and bifocal IOLs, zonal-progressive multifocal refractive lenses were developed. These simultaneous-vision lenses provide distance, intermediate, and near correction within the area of the ocular pupil. Recently, phakic multifocal IOLs have been designed and implanted, and a new foldable apodized diffractive IOL with unique optics in acrylic material has been produced.

Allergan Medical Optics Array and Allergan Medical Optics Rezoom Multifocal Intraocular Lenses

The first multifocal IOL to be approved by the United States FDA was the AMO Array multifocal IOL (Allergan, Irvine, Calif) (Model SI40N). The foldable AMO Array multifocal IOL has a series of repeatable, continual aspheric power distributions on the anterior surface of the lens (Figure 9-4). The power profile was designed to smooth the transitions between zones, diminishing the appearance of halos around light and allowing for a range of focus from far to near.

Relative or absolute contraindications include the presence of ocular pathologies that may degrade the image formation or may be associated with less than adequate visual function postoperatively despite the visual improvement following surgery. Exclusion criteria are: patients with monofocal IOL in the fellow eye, uncontrolled glaucoma, progressive diabetic retinopathy, age-related macular degeneration, recurrent inflammation, corneal lesions that may alter the visual acuity, preoperative astigmatism higher that 1.5 D, driving, and operations during the night.

A precise preoperative biometry and an accurate IOL power calculation, as well as a good surgical technique in selecting and positioning the lens, are crucial to reduce the incidence of complications

Figure 9-4 (Pearl 38). AMO Array Multifocal IOL has a series of repeatable, continual aspheric power distributions on its anterior surface.

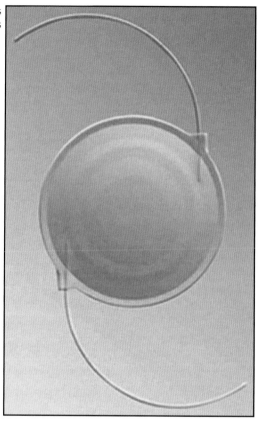

like IOL power miscalculation, decentration, and insufficient near vision acuity. A successful refractive outcome can be obtained with proper patient selection, motivation, and realistic expectations.

All trials report lower CS with the multifocal IOL, which is consistent with the expected optical effect of the lens. Montes-Mico et al showed that the Array multifocal IOL, with its center-distance design, is distance biased. Distance CS is within normal limits under bright photopic conditions but shows deficits at higher spatial frequencies under dim mesopic conditions. For all spatial frequencies and illumination conditions, near CS obtained with the multifocal IOL is below that which can be achieved by an appropriate monofocal near correction.

Complications of surgery can be expected to be similar for multifocal and monofocal IOLs because the lenses are similar in all but the design of the optics and require no modifications to surgical technique.

The recently FDA-approved Rezoom multifocal hydrophobic acrylic IOL (Model NXG1), from AMO (Allergan, Irvine, Calif), has a 6-mm optic with five concentric refractive zones: zones 1, 3, and 5 are distance dominant; zones 2 and 4 are near dominant; and an aspheric transition among zones provides balanced intermediate vision. It has an optic edge design (Optiedge design [AMO Inc, Santa Anna, Calif]) to minimize lens epithelial cell migration and the intensity of reflected images and edge glare. This lens seems to provide good distance vision and satisfactory intermediate and near vision under different light conditions.

In a study comparing both models, the Rezoom lens had superior outcomes in several aspects. The mean defocus acuity curves for both IOLs were similar; they demonstrated acceptable near vision and excellent intermediate vision. All study patients with the Rezoom lens reported that they can function comfortably without glasses at distance (100%), intermediate (95%), and near (71%). Sixty-seven percent of patients did not wear glasses for all distances 6 months postoperatively. All patients reported that they could easily drive a car.

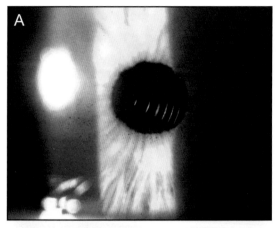

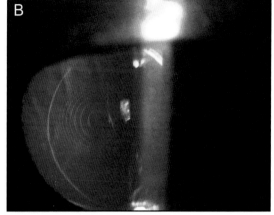

Figure 9-5 (Pearl 38). Decentered ReSTOR IOL secondary to anterior capsular capture of the optic edge seen (A) before and (B) after pupillary dilation. (C) Repositioning of the IOL was performed within 1 week of the initial surgery. (Courtesy of Samir A. Melki, MD, PhD.)

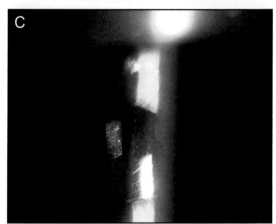

Distance-corrected near visual acuity was 20/40 or better in 83.3% of patients. Mean binocular uncorrected distance VA was 20/20. Mean uncorrected near visual acuity at 40 cm was 20/42, and distance-corrected VA at 40 cm was 20/35. Binocular best-corrected distance VA was 20/25 and better in all eyes. Compared to the Array IOL, the Rezoom IOL produced fewer photic phenomena (eg, halos, glare, and starbursts). Specifically, the incidence of halos was one-third that with the Array lens. This lens was approved using European data and as an upgrade to the Array Multifocal IOL.

Alcon RESTOR Multifocal Intraocular Lens

In March 2005, this new multifocal IOL was approved by the FDA. The multicenter FDA United States clinical trial results for more than 500 patients is now available. The Acrysof ReSTOR IOL (Alcon Laboratories Inc, Forth Worth, Tex) has an apodized diffractive optic technology. This lens is available in both a multi-piece (MA6OD3) and single-piece (SA6OD3) (Figure 9-5) design with the optics on hydrophobic acrylic. The asymmetric biconvex design features a 13 mm overall diameter (6.0 mm optic diameter) with an apodized diffractive pattern in the central region of the anterior surface of the optic. Hydrophobic acrylic (single-piece) or PMMA (multi-piece) haptics secure the lens within the capsular bag.

The FDA US Clinical Trial for this IOL showed well-satisfied patients, minimal visual symptoms, and few social limitations together with good near and distance visual acuities. Cumulative binocular photopic distance-corrected near visual acuity was 20/40 or better (J3) in about 98% and 20/25 or better (J1) in about 77% of patients. Binocular uncorrected near VA was 20/25 or better (J1) in about 72%. Cumulative binocular photopic uncorrected distance VA was 20/20 or better in about 60% and 20/40

Figure 9-6 (Pearl 38). Alcon Acrylic platform IOLs may not always center correctly despite adequate placement in the capsular bag. Transillumination view of an SAGOAT IOL in a patient with Albinism illustrates this point. This could be due to a centration mismatch between the capsular bag and the pupil. (Courtesy of Samir A. Melki, MD, PhD.)

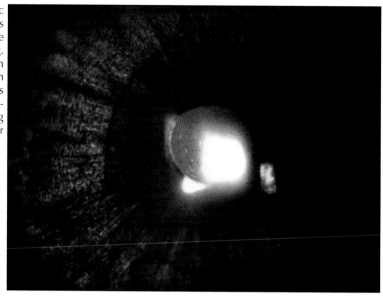

or better in almost 100% of patients. Binocular best-corrected distance VA was 20/20 or better in 89% and 20/25 or better in all patients. However, some limitations have to be considered when planning to use this IOL. The FDA study showed that monocular implanted patients had worse distance UCVA and BCVA and had more night vision problems, glare, and haloes compared to patients implanted with the monofocal control IOL. Among the bilaterally implanted patients, the improvement in distance-corrected near vision was greater under photopic than mesopic conditions. Mean spherical add power needed to achieve BCVA for near was higher under mesopic conditions (mean value of 2.5 D) than photopic conditions (range of mean values: 0.09 to 0.16 D). Older subjects implanted with the AcrySof ReSTOR lens (eg, >80 years old) demonstrated a trend for poorer distance UCVA than the monofocal controls. At an intermediate distance of 70 cm, the percentage of eyes achieving 20/20 or better UCVA and 20/25 or better distance BCVA was significantly worse for the ReSTOR IOL as compared to the monofocal control. For binocular CS at 12 and 18 cycles per degree, the percentage of ReSTOR patients able to see at least one grating ranged from 85.9% to 75% compared to 95.8% to 90.6% of monofocal control patients. Finally, a night driving simulation test showed that under glare conditions, the ability of ReSTOR patients to identify text signs was reduced on average by 28%. Apart from these limitations, ReSTOR IOL spectacle independence rates were statistically better (around 80%) (p < 0.0001) than control rates (7.7%) and satisfaction scores without glasses were also significantly better (p = 0.0029) than controls.

The ReSTOR IOL is a single piece acrylic lens of similar make-up to the SA60-AT platform. Figure 9-6 illustrates how those lenses can be decentered relative to the pupil entrance despite adequate in-the-bag placement. This can be due to either centration mismatch between the capsular bag and the pupil or to the failure to manually center the IOL at the end of surgery. To avoid decentration of multifocal single-piece acrylic IOL such as the ReSTOR lens, we recommend aligning the central ring on fixation by asking the patient to look at the microscope light at the end of surgery. It seems that these lenses will remain in the position in which they are left at the end of the procedure.

A mismatch may sometimes be noted between the pupillary center and the single piece acrylic multifocal IOL despite the above measures. This is most likely due to a decentered pupil. Figure 9-6 illustrates this point in a transillumination view of a single-piece acrylic monofocal IOL (SA60-AT) adequately placed in the capsular bag.

IOLTECH Newlife/Vivarte Phakic Multifocal Intraocular Lens

Vivarte Presbyopic phakic refractive lens (PRL), now called Newlife (IOLTECH, SA, La Rochelle, France), is a three-point anterior chamber angle-supported phakic lens with multifocal optics. It has a 5.5-mm optic with three concentric refractive zones on the anterior face: one central 1.5-mm zone for distance vision, one 0.55-mm ring zone for near vision (with an addition of +2.50 D), and another 211.45-mm outer ring zone for distance vision. IOL power is available from –5 to +5 D by 0.5-D intervals. The optic is hydrophilic acrylic, while the haptics are made of PMMA with hydrophilic acrylic footplates. The IOL is foldable and can be injected through 3.2-mm incisions under topical anesthesia or peribulbar. In a recently published study by Baikoff et al, 55 eyes of 33 patients have been implanted and followed for 2 to 83 weeks. The initial refraction was between –5.00 D and +5.00 D. Exclusion criteria were shallow anterior chamber and low endothelial cell count. Postoperatively, the mean refraction was –0.12 ± 0.51 D, the mean decimal uncorrected distance acuity was 0.78 ± 0.20, and the mean Parinaud uncorrected near acuity was 2.3 ± 0.6. Eighty-four percent of eyes achieved an uncorrected distance acuity of 0.60 or better and an uncorrected near acuity of Parinaud 3 or better. However, patients experienced a mean one-line loss in best-corrected distance visual acuity, the occurrence of halos (24%), pupil ovalization (10%), and endothelial cell loss (5%) 1 year after surgery. Four IOLs (7.27%) had to be explanted because patients were not satisfied with the results. A multifocal phakic IOL is a permanent yet reversible treatment option for presbyopia. This approach will probably be incorporated in other phakic IOLs in the near future.

Always Remember…

Multifocal and accommodative IOLs are still in their infancy. Future advances will be needed before widespread acceptance.

Ensure precise multifocal lens centration at the end of surgery.

BIBLIOGRAPHY

Acrysof ReSTOR FDA Summary of Safety and Effectiveness Data. Available at: http://www.fda.gov/cdrh/pdf4/p040020b.pdf. Accessed on 06/13/2005.

Alio JL, Tavolato M, De la Hoz F, et al. Near vision restoration with refractive lens exchange and pseudoaccommodating and multifocal refractive and diffractive intraocular lenses Comparative clinical study. *J Cataract Refract Surg.* 2004;30(12):2494-2503.

Baikoff G, Matach G, Fontaine A, Ferraz C, Spera C. Correction of presbyopia with refractive multifocal phakic intraocular lenses. *J Cataract Refract Surg.* 2004;30(7):1454-1460.

Bissen-Miyajima H. Multifocal IOLs for presbyopia. In: Tsubota K, Boxer Wachler BS, Azar DT, Koch DD, eds. *Hyperopia and Presbyopia.* New York, NY: Marcel Dekker Ltd; 2003.

Buehl W, Findl O, Menapace R, et al. Effect of an acrylic intraocular lens with a sharp posterior optic edge on posterior capsule opacification. *J Cataract Refract Surg.* 2002;28:1105-1111.

Charters L. How to evaluate presbyopic patients for monovision. *Ophthalmology Times.* 2000;(25):109.

Claoue C. Functional vision after cataract removal with multifocal and accommodating intraocular lens implantation: prospective comparative evaluation of Array multifocal and 1CU accommodating lenses. *J Cataract Refract Surg.* 2004;30(10):2088-2091.

Coren S, Kaplan CP. Patterns of ocular dominance. *Am J Optom Arch Acad Optom.* 1973;(50):283-292.

Cumming JS, Slade SG, Chayet A. Clinical evaluation of the model AT-45 silicone accommodating intraocular lens: results of feasibility and the initial phase of a Food and Drug Administration clinical trial. *Ophthalmology.* 2001;108(11):2005-2009; discussion 2010.

Cumming JS. The accommodating intraocular lens. In: Agarwal A, ed. *Presbyopia: A Surgical Textbook.* Thorofare, NJ: SLACK Incorporated; 2002.

Dick B. Assessment of three accommodative IOLs. *Cataract and Refractive Surgery Today.* 2004;July:56-57.

Dick HB. Experience with the Rezoom IOL. Comparing this lens with the Array. *Cataract Refract Surg Today.* 2005. Available at: http://www.crstoday.com/PDF%20Articles/0605/CRST0605_F11_Dick.html. Accessed September 27, 2005.

Dolders MG, Nijkamp MD, Nuijts RM, et al. Cost effectiveness of foldable multifocal intraocular lenses compared to foldable monofocal intraocular lenses for cataract surgery. *Br J Ophthalmol.* 2004;88(9):1163-1168.

Ellingson FT. Explantation of 3M diffractive intraocular lenses. *J Cataract Refract Surg.* 1990;16(6):697-702.

Ellis MF. Sharp-edged intraocular lens design as a cause of permanent glare. *J Cataract Refract Surg.* 2001;27:1061-1064.

Fernandez-Suntany JP, Pineda Rn, Azar DT. Conductive keratoplasty. *Int Ophthalmol Clin.* 2004;44(1):161-168.

Franchini A, Gallarti BZ, Vaccari E. Computerized analysis of the effects of intraocular lens edge design on the quality of vision in pseudophakic patients. *J Cataract Refract Surg.* 2003;29:342-347.

Fukasaku H, Marron JA. Anterior ciliary sclerotomy with silicone expansion plug implantation: effect on presbyopia and intraocular pressure. *Int Ophthalmol Clin.* 2001;41(2):133-141.

Gimbel HV, Sanders DR, Raanan MG. Visual and refractive results of multifocal intraocular lenses. *Ophthalmology.* 1991;98(6):881-887; discussion 888.

Glasser A, Kaufman PL. The mechanism of accommodation in primates. *Ophthalmology.* 1999;106(5):863-872.

Goldberg DB. Comparison of myopes and hyperopes after laser in situ keratomileusis monovision. *J Cataract Refract Surg.* 2003;29(9):1695-1701.

Hamilton DR, Davidorf JM, Maloney RK. Anterior ciliary sclerotomy for treatment of presbyopia: a prospective controlled study. *Ophthalmology.* 2002;109(11):1970-1976; discussion 1976-1977.

Helmholtz HV. Handbuch der physiologishen optik. In: Southall JPC, ed. *Helmholtz's Treatise on Physiological Optics.* New York, NY: Dover Publications; 1962:143–172.

Ian S, Glasser A. Evaluation of a satisfied bilateral scleral expansion band patient. *J Cataract Refract Surg.* 2004;30(7):1445-1453.

Ito M, Asano-Kato N, Fukagawa K, Arai H, Toda I, Tsubota K. Ocular integrity after anterior ciliary sclerotomy and scleral ablation by the Er:YAG laser. *J Refract Surg.* 2005;21(1):77-81.

Jain S, Arora I, Azar DT. Success of monovision in presbyopes: review of the literature and potential applications to refractive surgery. *Surv Ophthalmol.* 1996;40(6):491-499.

Jay JL, Chakrabarti HS, Morrison JD. Quality of vision through diffractive bifocal intraocular lenses. *Br J Ophthalmol.* 1991;75(6):359-366.

Klein S, Fry K, Hersh PS. Laser in situ keratomileusis after conductive keratoplasty. *J Cataract Refract Surg.* 2004;30(3):702-705.

Kuchle M, Nguyen NX, Langenbucher A, et al. Implantation of a new accommodative posterior chamber intraocular lens. *J Refract Surg.* 2002;18(3):208-216.

Kuchle M, Nguyen NX, Langenbucher A, et al. Two years experience with the new accommodative 1CU intraocular lens. *Ophthalmologe.* 2002;99(11):820-824.

Kymionis GD, Aslanides M, Khoury AN, et al. Laser in situ keratomileusis for residual hyperopic astigmatism after conductive keratoplasty. *J Refract Surg.* 2004;20(3):276-278.

Kymionis GD, Naoumidi TL, Aslanides IM, Pallikaris IG. Corneal iron ring after conductive keratoplasty. *Am J Ophthalmol.* 2003;136(2):378-379.

Kymionis GD, Titze P, Markomanolakis MM, et al. Corneal perforation after conductive keratoplasty with previous refractive surgery. *J Cataract Refract Surg.* 2003;29(12):2452-2454.

Leyland M, Zinicola E. Multifocal versus monofocal intraocular lenses in cataract surgery: a systematic review. *Ophthalmology.* 2003;110(9):1789-1798.

Lin DY, Manche EE. Two-year results of conductive keratoplasty for the correction of low to moderate hyperopia. *J Cataract Refract Surg.* 2003;29(12):2339-2350.

Lin JT, Mallo O. Treatment of presbyopia by infrared laser radial sclerectomy. *J Refract Surg.* 2003;19(4):465-467.

Malecaze FJ, Gazagne CS, Tarroux MC, Gorrand JM. Scleral expansion bands for presbyopia. *Ophthalmology.* 2001;108(12):2165-2171.

Mastropasqua L, Toto L, Nubile M, Falconio G, Ballone E. Clinical study of the 1CU accommodating intraocular lens. *J Cataract Refract Surg.* 2003;29(7):1307-1312.

Mathews S. Scleral expansion surgery does not restore accommodation in human presbyopia. *Ophthalmology.* 1999;106(5):873-877.

McDonald MB, Davidorf J, Maloney RK, et al. Conductive keratoplasty for the correction of low to moderate hyperopia: 1-year results on the first 54 eyes. *Ophthalmology.* 2002;109(4):637-649.

McDonald MB, Hersh PS, Manche EE, et al. Conductive keratoplasty for the correction of low to moderate hyperopia: US clinical trial 1-year results on 355 eyes. *Ophthalmology.* 2002;109:1978-1989.

McGill EC, Erickson P. Sighting dominance and monovision distance binocular fusional ranges. *J Am Optom Assoc.* 1991;62(10):738-742.

McLeod SD, Portney V, Ting A. A dual optic accommodating foldable intraocular lens. *Br J Ophthalmol.* 2003;87(9):1083-1085.

Miranda D, Krueger RR. Monovision laser in situ keratomileusis for pre-presbyopic and presbyopic patients. *J Refract Surg.* 2004;20(4):325-328.

Montes-Mico R, Alio JL. Distance and near contrast sensitivity function after multifocal intraocular lens implantation. *J Cataract Refract Surg.* 2003;29(4):703-711.

Nijkamp MD, Dolders MG, de Brabander J, et al. Effectiveness of multifocal intraocular lenses to correct presbyopia after cataract surgery: a randomized controlled trial. *Ophthalmology.* 2004;111(10):1832-1839.

Ostrin LA, Kasthurirangan S, Glasser A. Evaluation of a satisfied bilateral scleral expansion band patient. *J Cataract Refract Surg.* 2004;30(7):1445-1453.

Pineda-Fernandez A, Jaramillo J, Celis V, et al. Refractive outcomes after bilateral multifocal intraocular lens implantation. *J Cataract Refract Surg.* 2004;30(3):685-688.

Probst L. The C&C Vision CrystaLens model AT-45 silicone intraocular lens. In: Agarwal A, ed. *Presbyopia: A Surgical Textbook.* Thorofare, NJ: SLACK Incorporated; 2002:201.

Qazi MA, Pepose JS, Shuster JJ. Implantation of scleral expansion band segments for the treatment of presbyopia. *Am J Ophthalmol.* 2002;134(6):808-815.

Sacu S, Menapace R, Buehl W, et al. Effect of intraocular lens optic edge design and material on fibrotic capsule opacification and capsulorhexis contraction. *J Cataract Refract Surg.* 2004;30:1875-1882.

Schachar RA, Huang T, Huang X. Mathematic proof of Schachar's hypothesis of accommodation. *Ann Ophthalmol.* 1993;25(1):5-9.

Schachar RA. Presbyopic surgery. *Int Ophthalmol Clin.* 2002;42(4):107-118.

Schachar RA. The correction of presbyopia. *Int Ophthalmol Clin.* 2001;41(2):53-70.

Schor C, Erickson P. Patterns of binocular suppression and accommodation in monovision. *Am J Optom Physiol Opt.* 1988;65(11):853-861.

Schor C, Landsman L, Erickson P. Ocular dominance and the interocular suppression of blur in monovision. *Am J Optom Physiol Opt.* 1987;64(10):723-730.

Sen HN, Sarikkola AU, Uusitalo RJ, Laatikainen L. Quality of vision after AMO Array multifocal intraocular lens implantation. *J Cataract Refract Surg.* 2004;30(12):2483-2493.

Sippel KC, Jain S, Azar DT. Monovision achieved with excimer laser refractive surgery. *Int Ophthalmol Clin.* 2001;41(2):91-101.

Thornton, SP, Shear NA. *Surgery for Hyperopia and Presbyopia.* Baltimore, Md: Williams & Wilkins; 1997.

Werner L, Pandey SK, Izak AM, et al. Capsular bag opacification after experimental implantation of a new accommodating intraocular lens in rabbit eyes. *J Cataract Refract Surg.* 2004;30:1114-1123.

Wright KW, Guemes A, Kapadia MS, Wilson SE. Binocular function and patient satisfaction after monovision induced by myopic photorefractive keratectomy. *J Cataract Refract Surg.* 1999;25(2):177-182.

CHAPTER 10

SEVEN
PEARLS IN PHAKIC INTRAOCULAR
LENS IMPLANTATION

Thanh Hoang-Xuan, MD; Jean-Louis Arné, MD; and Georges Baikoff, MD

The last several years have witnessed an increased interest in phakic IOLs as the limitations of corneal refractive surgery have become clear. The rapid development of new phakic IOL designs has led to significant improvements in the safety for the procedure. However, widespread acceptance and United States regulatory approval are still pending because each lens still suffers from limitations related to concerns of corneal endothelial cells or lenticular damage. This chapter presents several pearls related to the implantation of anterior chamber, iris-fixated, and posterior chamber phakic IOLs.

PEARL #39: PHAKIC INTRAOCULAR LENSES: WHAT SIZE?

One of the most important preoperative considerations for phakic IOL implantation is the determination of IOL size. For the Nuvita Baikoff anterior chamber phakic IOL (Figure 10-1), determination of lens size relies on the measurement of the horizontal white-to-white distance using surgical compass calipers and best done under the operating microscope. The implant size is calculated by adding 0.5 mm to the white-to-white distance if the anterior chamber is not deep. In deep anterior chamber angles, one should add up to but not more than 1 mm to the measured distance. New devices that allow accurate measurement of the internal diameter of the anterior chamber are under development and may obviate the need to perform such calculations. For the Verisyse iris-claw phakic IOL (Ophtec, Boca Raton, Fla), there is a single haptic-to-haptic size of 8.5 mm (Figures 10-2A and 10-2B). This is one of the advantages of this implant over the angle-supported and posterior chamber phakic IOLs. However, the surgeon has the choice between two diameters of the optic: 5 mm and 6 mm.

For the STAAR collamer posterior chamber phakic IOL (STAAR Surgical, Monrovia, Calif) (Figure 10-3), there is a theoretical correspondence between the white-to-white distance and the overall length of the ICL. For myopic eyes, the size of the ICL must be equal to the white-to-white measurement, +0.5 to 0.6 mm rounded to the nearest 0.5-mm increment. In the event of an intermediate value, the larger diameter must be chosen, but the difference must always be lower than 0.9 mm. For hyperopic eyes, the length of the ICL must be equal to the white-to-white measurement rounded to the superior available size. If the ICL is too short for the sulcus, the lens vault may be insufficient to clear the crystalline lens, exposing it to the risk of an anterior capsular cataract. If it is too long, the lens will vault excessively, crowding the angle and possibly causing closed-angle glaucoma. An ideal vault is 500 μm over the crystalline lens.

Always Remember...

The Verisyse phakic IOL has a single size: 8.5 mm.

Gross measurement of horizontal white-to-white distance is not accurate enough for adequate sizing of the Nuvita and the STAAR lenses.

Figure 10-1 (Pearl 39). The Nuvita phakic IOL. (Courtesy of Bausch & Lomb Surgical.)

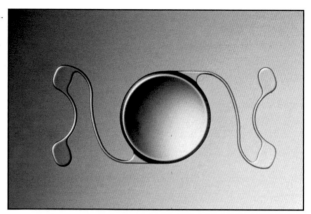

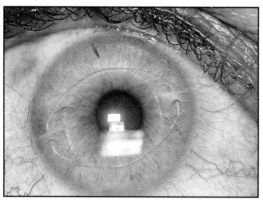

Figure 10-2A (Pearl 39). The Artisan iris-claw phakic IOL. (Courtesy of OPHTEC.)

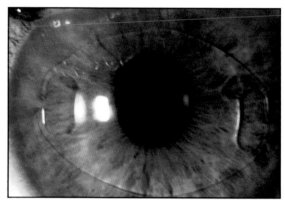

Figure 10-2B (Pearl 39). The Verisyse Artisan iris-claw phakic IOL.

Figure 10-3 (Pearl 39). The STAAR PC phakic IOL; ICL. (Courtesy of Bausch & Lomb Surgical.)

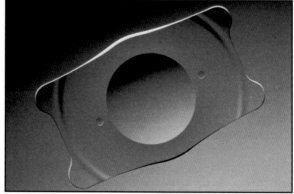

Pearl #40: Iris Visco-Stretch Prevents Mydriasis and Iris Prolapse

Iris prolapse is an event that may jeopardize anterior chamber and Verisyse IOL implantation into phakic eyes and usually results from viscoelastic material going under the iris. Reinserting the prolapsed iris is very difficult, and a peripheral iridectomy is usually not sufficient to let the viscoelastic material escape out of the posterior chamber unless it is very large. Also, repetitive instrumental maneuvers will rapidly provoke iris pigment epithelium dispersion and iris atrophy. A vicious circle occurs if viscoelastic material is introduced into the eye at this stage—the more viscoelastic that is injected, the more the prolapse.

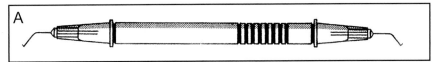

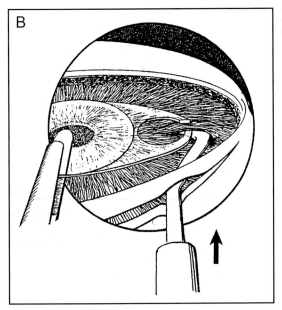

Figure 10-4 (Pearl 41). (A) Iris enclavation: a specially designed needle. (B) Iris enclavation: the needle is used to fold the iris enclavate between the claws of the Artisan lens. (Courtesy of OPHTEC.)

Precise handling of the viscoelastic material is required. At the beginning of the procedure, do not inject too much viscoelastic material into the eye, just the amount necessary to perform the corneal incisions. Just after the incisions have been performed, viscoelastic material is injected over the iris at 12 o'clock and is pushed against the lens. The anterior chamber is then filled progressively with the viscoelastic material. The iris near the incision should be observed throughout the procedure. Viscoelastic is added onto the iris base as soon as the iris starts to bulge forward. The injection of viscoelastics is best performed with the tip of the cannula close to the iris in order to induce iris stretching centripetally and the tendency of the viscoelastic material to pass under the iris. Iris visco-stretch can also reverse intraoperative mydriasis due to the passage of the viscoelastic material through the pupil. Iris manipulation in this manner will facilitate iris enclavation of Verisyse lenses.

Always Remember...

> *Stretch the iris centripetally with the viscoelastic material as soon as the iris bulges forward or the pupil starts to dilate.*

> *Intraoperative iris prolapse may be due to excessive viscoelastic material in the eye.*

PEARL #41: VERISYSE LENS: IRIS ENCLAVATION

Perhaps the most difficult step of Verisyse phakic IOL implantation is iris enclavation into the Artisan's claws (Figure 10-4). Specially designed disposable enclavation needles are provided by the manufacturer to make a fold at the midperiphery of the iris, but the location, size, and direction of the two port incisions are critical to achieving this goal and centering the lens properly. If the incisions are not properly performed, corneal folds will be induced, preventing visualization of the surgical maneuvers, which may lead to poor IOL fixation and/or decentration.

Figure 10-5 (Pearl 41). Paracentesis incisions should be created parallel (left) rather than radial (right) to the limbus to prevent corneal striae during surgical manipulation with the enclavation needle.

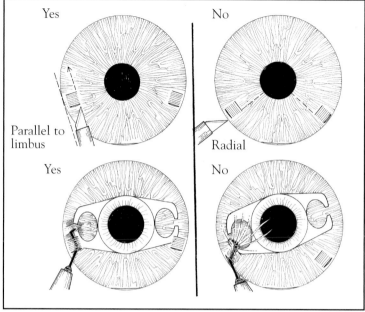

The port incisions should be performed in a manner different from those during cataract surgery, in which the standard paracentesis is directed radially. The blade should enter the cornea 1 clock hour above the meridian of enclavation, next to the limbal arcades, and enter the anterior chamber about 1 mm from the limbus and just above the (horizontal or vertical) meridian of enclavation (Figure 10-5). The size of the port incisions should be about 1.5 mm. This allows for adequate manipulation of the iris enclavation needles vertically without inducing corneal folds. In addition, disenclavation maneuvers will be facilitated using this approach.

Always Remember...

Port incisions parallel to the limbus provide better comfort for iris enclavation maneuvers.

PEARL #42: IMPLANTABLE CONTACT LENS: PREVENT PIGMENT DISPERSION

Pigment deposition on the surface of an implantable contact lens (ICL) has no visual consequences, but pigmentary deposits in the angle can be of some concern because highly myopic patients are, by their nature, at increased risk of developing glaucoma. Pigment dispersion can be minimized by avoiding the dialing technique of implantation. This technique involves rotating the implant 180 degrees after positioning the distal footplates in the posterior chamber and the surgeon placing the others footplates in nasal position. Even if the manipulations are smooth and gentle, trauma to the posterior iris pigment epithelium may occur. A nonrotational technique is advisable to avoid pigment dispersion. The distal haptics are inserted first; the micromanipulator is inserted in the anterior chamber through the main incision. A light downward pressure is applied to push the haptics under the iris. The manipulator is then reintroduced through the side port, and the proximal haptics are placed beneath the iris.

A surgical iridectomy is preferred over preoperative YAG iridotomies, which induce pigment dispersion. The surgical iridectomy is performed perpendicular to the longitudinal axis of the ICL to exclude the risk of occlusion by the haptics. The ICL is placed horizontally (at 3 and 9 o'clock), and the iridectomy is situated between 10 and 2 o'clock. A forceps with fine teeth is introduced into the anterior chamber through a vertical corneal incision. The iris is caught close to the base, and using iris scissors, the iridectomy is performed. Some surgeons prefer performing the iridectomy with a vitrector at the beginning of surgery (before dilating the pupil). Mydriasis is obtained by an infusion of epinephrine into the anterior chamber.

Preoperative YAG laser iridotomies are best performed in two different locations. We use two double-burst of 7.0 milli-joules in an iris crypt around the 11 and 1 o'clock positions.

Always Remember…

Thrusting the footplates behind the iris using a small injection of viscoelastic substance can facilitate ICL positioning. After cutting the iris, a fine cannula must be inserted through the corneal incision followed by gentle aspiration of the pigment.

PEARL #43: THE INVERTED IMPLANTABLE CONTACT LENS

As may happen during cataract surgery, the posterior chamber IOL may become inverted during insertion. This is not common during ICL surgery, but the prevention and management approach is important. The surgeon must never try to overturn the ICL inside the anterior chamber. After cataract extraction, there is 8 or 9 mm of working space from the corneal endothelium to the posterior capsule, but in ICL surgery, the space from the endothelium to the anterior capsule is only 3.5 mm. Despite the presence of viscoelastic material, a maneuver to overturn the implant may cause irreversible damage to the crystalline lens and to the endothelium. Removing the implant and repeating the procedure is preferable. The removal technique is relatively simple: viscoelastic is injected below and above the implant; the incision is extended to 3.5 mm; the proximal footplate is caught using a forceps with smooth polished jaws, and the lens is gently pulled; then, a second forceps placed tangentially to the limbus grasps the haptic as the lens is pulled outward. This maneuver is repeated until one-third of the implant is outside the eye. The ICL is then extracted in one movement. To avoid damaging the ICL optic and to allow its reinsertion, the forceps should not come into contact with the central zone.

Using folding forceps rather than a lens injector will minimize the risk of ICL inversion. Although the use of an injector allows a small incision, it is very difficult to control the unfolding of the ICL. The forceps technique provides the surgeon with better control throughout the procedure: the implant is folded lengthwise using MacPherson forceps; the tip of the forceps is introduced in the entrance of the tunnel; another MacPherson forceps is then taken in the other hand and grabs the side of the implant; the first forceps is opened, and it regrasps the implant a little further and pushes it slowly. By alternating the implant movement into the tunnel, the tip of the forceps does not enter the anterior chamber. With this technique, the surgeon can check the orientation of the implant and avoid an inverted ICL.

Always Remember…

The central part of a myopic ICL is the thinnest, and only a thin layer of viscoelastic separates it from the anterior capsule during surgery. The lens epithelial cells have no repair ability; thus, surgical trauma leads to lens opacification.

PEARL #44: REMOVAL OF THE VISCOELASTIC AGENT

During phakic IOL surgery, most surgeons use a cohesive viscoelastic material. Complete removal of the viscoelastic is an important step at the end of the surgery.

In the case of posterior phakic IOLs, viscoelastics must be removed completely. The presence of residual viscoelastic material trapped behind the implant may cause opacification of the crystalline lens. As soon as the haptics are in position behind the iris and while the pupil is still dilated, gentle infusion of balanced salt solution is performed with a cannula through the main incision, which forces the viscoelastic material out of the posterior chamber. This is followed by using an irrigation/aspiration (I/A) manual cannula to complete removal of the viscoelastic agent. The aspiration tip may have to reach behind the ICL, passing lateral to the optic. A miotic agent is then injected, and the aspiration is completed. The infusion flow must be perfectly regulated in order to avoid overfilling or flattening the anterior chamber.

In the case of anterior chamber phakic IOLs and iris-fixated IOLs, the cannula is introduced into the anterior chamber at 6 o'clock, and balanced salt solution is injected. A slight depression of these lenses and of the inferior lip of the incision will ascertain complete removal. An I/A cannula may be used if needed. Some surgeons prefer a bimanual I/A technique for thorough viscoelastic removal.

Always Remember...

Meticulous removal of the viscoelastic agent at the end of phakic IOL surgery is very important, especially for posterior chamber phakic IOLs.

Pearl #45: Bioptics

"Bioptics" is a word which was invented by Zaldivar to describe the implantation of a posterior chamber hydrogel-collagen plate phakic IOL (STAAR Collamer ICL) followed by LASIK surgery to treat extreme myopia. Definition of bioptics can be expanded to the combination of any corneal refractive procedure (LASIK, PRK, LASEK, or even intracorneal ring segments [Intacs]) not only to all types of phakic IOLs (PRL, Artisan iris-claw lens, or angle-supported phakic IOLs), but also to clear lensectomy or pseudophakic surgery to treat high ametropia with astigmatism. The timing of the corneal refractive procedure is variable, depending on the type of the intraocular surgery. When an anterior chamber phakic IOL is implanted as part as a bioptics procedure, it is strongly recommended to perform the lamellar microkeratome cut during the same procedure, before lens insertion, in order to prevent IOL-corneal endothelial touch during the cut. In case of phakic IOL implantation, the inclusion criteria (anterior chamber depth, corneal endothelial cell density, and pupil size) must be fulfilled.

The main indication of bioptics is the correction of refractive errors that are beyond the treatment range of current IOL designs; then, the residual spherical and/or cylindrical ametropia is treated with LASIK or PRK/LASEK. Toric phakic anterior (Artiflex) and posterior (ICL) chamber IOLs are currently available in certain countries, allowing some "debulk" of the astigmatic error.

Because successful refractive surgery depends as much on quality of vision as on refractive efficacy, it is of highest importance to select the most optimal combination of power ranges to treat with the two respective procedures of bioptics. The higher the ametropia to treat, the smaller the effective optical zone and the higher the induction of glare and halos, especially in dim illumination conditions and when the pupil is large. Thus bioptics strategy, by splitting the refractive error between the two procedures, will better prevent or reduce these complications than corneal refractive surgery or phakic IOL implantation alone. It is useful to know that Verisyse phakic iris-claw lenses are available with optical zones of 6 mm for myopic power ranges of 15 D and below.

Always Remember...

Differentiate between corneal and refractive astigmatism for better surgical planning in bioptics surgery.

Bibliography

Arné JL, Lesueur LC. Phakic posterior chamber lenses for high myopia: functional and anatomical outcomes. *J Cataract Refract Surg.* 2000;26:369-374.

Asseto V, Benedetti S, Pesando P. Collamer intraocular contact lens to correct high myopia. *J Cataract Refract Surg.* 1996;22:551-556.

Davidorf JM, Zaldivar R, Oscherow S. Posterior chamber phakic intraocular lens for hyperopia of +4 to +11 diopters. *J Refract Surg.* 1998;14:306-311.

Fechner PU, Haubitz I, Wichmann W, Wulff K. Worst-Fechner biconcave minus power phakic iris-claw lens. *J Refract Surg.* 1999;15:93-105.

Fechner PU, Singh D, Wulff K. Iris-claw lens in phakic eyes to correct hyperopia: preliminary study. *J Cataract Refract Surg.* 1998;24:48-56.

Fechner PU, van der Heijde GL, Worst JGF. The correction of myopia by lens implantation into phakic eyes. *Am J Ophthalmol.* 1989;107:659-663.

Finks AM, Gore C, Rosen E. Cataract development after implantation of the Staar Collamer posterior chamber phakic lens. *J Cataract Refract Surg.* 1999;25:278-282.

Kim DY, Reinstein DZ, Silverman RH, et al. Very high frequency ultrasound analysis of a new phakic posterior chamber intraocular lens in situ. *Am J Ophthalmol.* 1998;125:725-729.

Marinho A, Neves MC, Pinto MC, Vaz F. Posterior chamber silicone phakic intraocular lens. *J Refract Surg.* 1997;13:219-222.

Menezo JL, Avino JA, Cisneros AL, et al. Iris-claw phakic intraocular lens for high myopia. *J Refract Surg.* 1997;13:545-555.

Menezo JL, Cisneros AL, Rodriguez-Salvador V. Endothelial study of iris-claw phakic lenses: four year follow-up. *J Cataract Refract Surg.* 1998;24:1039-1049.

Mertens E, Tassignon MJ. Detachment of iris-claw haptic after implantation of phakic Worst anterior chamber lens: case report. *Bull Soc Belge Ophtalmol.* 1998;268:19-22.

Pérez-Santonja JJ, Bueno JL, Zato MA. Surgical correction of high myopia in phakic eyes with Worst-Fechner myopia intraocular lenses. *J Refract Surg.* 1997;13:268-284.

Pérez-Santonja JJ, Iradier MT, Benitez del Castillo JM, Serrano JM, Zato MA. Chronic subclinical inflammation in phakic eyes with intraocular lenses to correct myopia. *J Cataract Refract Surg.* 1996;22:183-187.

Rosen E, Gore C. Staar Collamer posterior chamber phakic intraocular lens to correct myopia and hyperopia. *J Cataract Refract Surg.* 1998;24:596-606.

Trindade F, Pereira F. Cataract formation after posterior chamber phakic intraocular lens implantation. *J Cataract Refract Surg.* 1998;24:1661-1663.

Zaldivar R, Davidorf JM, Oscherow S. Posterior chamber phakic IOL for myopia of -8 to -19 diopters. *J Refract Surg.* 1998;14:294-305.

CHAPTER 11

THREE
PEARLS FOR SUCCESSFUL CATARACT
SURGERY USING TOPICAL ANESTHESIA

H. John Shammas, MD and Rania M. Shammas, MD

Topical anesthesia has become the most common form of analgesia for phacoemulsification cataract surgery. Besides the fact that the administration of topical anesthesia is rapid and painless, the main advantage of surgery without retrobulbar or peribulbar anesthesia is the elimination of potential complications associated with the insertion of a sharp needle behind the globe. These complications include retrobulbar hemorrhage, lid hematoma, optic nerve injury, ocular perforation, postoperative diplopia, and respiratory arrest. Topical anesthesia could also prevent potentially serious systemic side effects associated with diminishing or discontinuing oral anticoagulation prior to cataract surgery.

Performing cataract surgery under topical anesthesia requires careful patient selection and minor modifications in surgical technique.

PEARL #46: ANESTHESIA WITHOUT AKINESIA: WHAT IF THE EYE MOVES?

Performing cataract surgery under topical anesthesia may sound intimidating compared to the comforting control of akinesia. Eye movement is not always to the surgeon's disadvantage because the patient, when asked, may position the eye to allow better red reflex or field exposure.

Certain surgical steps require complete control of ocular motion. The eye must be held firm when creating the corneal incision and during the capsulorrhexis step, as unexpected eye movements may result in potentially serious complications such as an irregular/large incision or a torn capsular bag. Grabbing the sclera with a toothed forceps or using a dedicated fixation ring is usually enough to immobilize the globe. Once the phacoemulsification needle or the I/A cannulae is introduced, control of the patient's eye movement becomes easier to achieve, especially if a bimanual technique is used. The absence of akinesia does not add significant difficulty to the procedure.

Always Remember…

You may use the patient's ability to move his or her eye to your advantage, allowing more convenient positioning, better red reflex, and easier surgery. Head movement during surgery may be more problematic than eye movement.

PEARL #47: ENHANCING TOPICAL ANESTHESIA WITH ADJUNCTIVE MEASURES

The most common topical anesthetic used in ophthalmology is 1% tetracaine; however, its effect lasts a short period of time. More efficient topical anesthesia is obtained with nonpreserved lidocaine 2% or 4% (preservative-free). It is withdrawn from the ampule with a syringe and used as eye drops. A few drops are applied to both eyes while the patient is in the holding area and as the patient enters the operating room. Soaking the Murocel drain with Lidocaine 2% or 4% (the same compound used as eye drops at the beginning of the surgery) will prolong the effect of topical anesthesia. Lidocaine gel 2% has recently gained popularity and is as effective in reducing pain during surgery as the nonpreserved lidocaine drops. It is usually applied in the lower fornix 20 minutes prior to surgery, eliminating the need for multiple eye drop application. Applying lidocaine gel to the eyelids also relieves discomfort from the

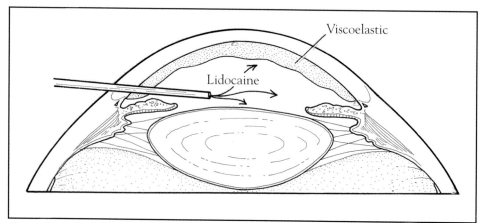

Figure 11-1 (Pearl 47). Viscoelastic material injected in the anterior chamber prior to lidocaine coats the corneal endothelium, preserving it from any potential toxic effect.

pressure of the speculum. A new viscous anesthetic eyedrop, TetraVisc (Ocusoft, Rosenberg, Tex), is now available. It works as well as the lidocaine jelly. It does not provide anesthesia to the lids but may be preferred by some surgeon because it is localized to the globe and avoids an oily surgical field.

Applying anesthetic eye drops or gel to the second eye will decrease lid squeezing and ocular movements in that eye, which in turn, results in fewer lid or eye movements in the operated eye.

Topical anesthesia may be supplemented by a small (0.1 cc) superior subconjunctival injection of the same nonpreserved lidocaine 2% or 4% if conjunctival manipulation is anticipated, including the insertion of a superior rectus bridle suture, conjunctival dissection, or the administration of subconjunctival antibiotics at the end of surgery. It is advisable to lift the conjunctiva with smooth forceps prior to the subconjunctival injection to avoid any bleeding.

Intraocular 1% lidocaine hydrochloride (HCL) can also be used as an adjunct to topical anesthesia. Although some surgeons use it routinely, it is mainly indicated in cases where the pupil does not fully dilate. Intraocular lidocaine decreases the pain and discomfort associated with iris manipulation during phacoemulsification or IOL insertion.

Sodium hyaluronate is first injected to avoid direct contact of the lidocaine with the corneal endothelium, protecting the endothelium from potential toxicity. Then, 0.1 to 0.2 ml of the unpreserved 1% lidocaine HCL is injected in the pupillary area (Figure 11-1). Intraocular lidocaine should not be used if the posterior capsule is compromised since retina and optic nerve damage may occur.

Patients undergoing cataract surgery are often anxious about the anticipated procedure. Some of them have a hard time holding still because of arthritic pains in the spine or the joints. Intravenous (IV) medications are very helpful in these instances. The most commonly used medications are midazolam HCL (midazolam) to relieve anxiety and provide sedation, and fentanyl citrate (fentanyl) for analgesia and sedation. If additional sedation is required, barbiturates such as sodium thiopental (Pentothal [Abbot Laboratories, Chicago, Ill]) or methohexital sodium (Brevital [Eli Lilly, Greenfield, Ind]) can be used in very low doses. A commonly used regimen for topical cataract surgery includes administration of 0.025 mg of fentanyl citrate when the patient is brought to the operating room. This is followed with 0.3 to 0.5 mg of midazolam HCL when surgery is ready to start. Additional doses are administered only when the need arises.

Patients may be frightened by unexpected colorful perceptions experienced during surgery. Informing the patient about possible visual sensations and talking to the patient in a soft, reassuring voice will alleviate a lot of the anxiety during the surgery and less IV medication will be needed.

Always Remember…

Apply topical anesthetic eye drops in the contralateral eye to decrease lid squeezing and ocular movement of both eyes.

Soaking the Murocel drain with lidocaine 2% or 4% (the same compound used as eye drops at the beginning of the surgery) will prolong the effect of topical anesthesia.

Do not use intraocular lidocaine during surgery if the integrity of the posterior capsule is compromised. Retina and optic nerve compromise may occur.

PEARL #48: THE UNSUITABLE CANDIDATE FOR TOPICAL ANESTHESIA

Not all patients can be safely operated on using topical anesthesia. Relative contraindications to topical anesthesia depend largely on the surgeon's confidence and ease of performing the phacoemulsification in a fast, efficient manner. Young patients are usually more anxious, and caution should be exercised when proceeding with topical anesthesia cataract surgery. Other warning signs have been called the Ds of disqualification:

- Difficult applanation tonometry (in the clinic)
- Deafness
- Degeneration (macula)
- Dysphagia, dyspnea
- Dementia
- Dense cataract
- Dysfunctional extraocular muscles (EOM)
- Drape phobia
- Difficulty during prior surgery
- Dilation difficulties (pupil)

Always Remember…

A previous complication during surgery in the contralateral eye is a relative contraindication to topical anesthesia.

BIBLIOGRAPHY

Bardocci A, Lofoco G, Perdicaro S, Ciucci F, Manna L. Lidocaine 2% gel versus lidocaine 4% unpreserved drops for topical anesthesia in cataract surgery. *Ophthalmology.* 2003;110:144-149.

Chong FC, Lai J, Lam D. Visual sensation during phacoemulsification and intraocular lens implantation using topical or regional anesthesia. *J Cataract Refract Surg.* 2004;30:444-448.

Jacobi PC, Dietlein TS, Jacobi FK. A comparative study of topical vs. retrobulbar anesthesia in complicated cataract surgery. *Arch Ophthalmol.* 2000;118(8):1037-1043.

Kirber WM. Lidocaine gel for topical anesthesia. *J Cataract Refract Surg.* 2000;26(2):163.

Quintyn JC, Calenda E, Retout A, Brasseur G. Topical anesthesia cataract surgery in patients with anticoagulant therapy. *J Cataract Refract Surg.* 2000;26(4):479-480.

Shammas HJ. Cataract surgery without retrobulbar or peribulbar anesthesia (letter). *J Cataract Refract Surg.* 1993;19:116.

Shammas HJ, Milkie M, Yeo R. Topical and subconjunctival anesthesia for phacoemulsification: prospective study. *J Cataract Refract Surg.* 1997;23:1577-1580.

8. Soliman M, Macky T, Samir K. Comparative clinical trial of topical anesthetic agents in cataract surgery. *J Cataract Refract Surg.* 2004;30:1716-1720.

9. Tan JH, Burton RL. Does preservative-free lignocaine 1% for hydrodissection reduce pain during phacoemulsification? *J Cataract Refract Surg.* 2000;26(5):733-735.

10. Yanguela J, Gomez-Arnau J, Martin-Rodrigo JC, et al. Diplopia after cataract surgery. *Ophthalmology.* 2004;111:686-692.

11. Yaylali V, Yildirim C, Tatlipinar S, et al. Subjective visual experiences and pain level during phacoemulsification and intraocular lens implantation under topical anesthesia. *Ophthalmologica.* 2003;217:413-416.

CHAPTER 12

FOUR
PEARLS TO CONQUER THE DIFFICULT IRIS

Pierre G. Mardelli, MD and Samir A. Melki, MD, PhD

We have all been faced with a "difficult iris" during cataract surgery. Usually an innocent bystander, an unruly iris may transform a routine case into a heart-throbbing experience with potentially dire outcomes. Adequate planning and a methodical approach are important in preventing and managing a rebellious iris.

PEARL #49: SMALL PUPIL, BIG CHALLENGE

With the chronic use of miotics, such as in long-standing glaucoma or in the presence of the pseudoexfoliation syndrome, the pupil may lose its elasticity and fail to dilate adequately for cataract surgery. A small pupil presents many challenges: small area for surgical maneuvers, poor red reflex, and difficulty to perform a continuous circular capsulorrhexis (CCC).

When anticipating surgery on a patient with a small pupil, the surgeon may resort to one or more of the following strategies to ensure surgical success: adequate pharmacological dilation, use of appropriate viscoelastics, iris stretching, use of iris hooks, and use of multiple microsphincterotomies.

Pharmacologic dilation can be enhanced using phenylephrine 10% if the blood pressure allows it. A combination of tropicamide 1%, cyclopentolate 1%, phenylephrine 2.5%, and a nonsteroidal anti-inflammatory agent may also be helpful. The use of intracameral epinephrine (1:10,000) may also be tried but is by no means a panacea. The use of epinephrine in the balanced salt solution bottle is helpful in keeping the pupil adequately dilated during the procedure.

Small pupils are often associated with posterior synechiae. Moving the tip of a viscoelastic cannula sideways can break these. The use of a retentive viscoelastic such as Viscoat (Alcon Surgical, Fort Worth, Tex) or Healon GV (Pharmacia Ophthalmics, Monrovia, Calif) allows manipulation of the iris with little trauma to the corneal endothelium and keeps the anterior chamber well formed. One should avoid injection of excessive viscoelastic material in the posterior chamber in order to allow greater pupillary dilation once the adhesions are released. Viscoelastics may also be used to dilate a medium-sized pupil or to aid in dilating the pupil after performing microsphincterectomies. The latter are usually created at the beginning of the case. After placing the viscoelastic, long Vannas scissors are used to make small cuts in the iris (usually three to five, inferiorly, nasally, and temporally). Viscoelastic material is reinjected to enlarge the pupil. If this is not sufficient, then stretching with the push-pull hooks may be helpful.

If the desired pupil size is not achieved with pharmacologic dilatation or viscoelastic manipulation, iris stretching may be useful. Stretching the iris is best performed with the help of a pair of push-pull or boat hooks (manufactured by many companies including Storz and Duckworth & Kent). These instruments are rounded on their lower edge and should not cause any damage to the anterior capsule. Fill the anterior chamber with viscoelastic material in an attempt to enlarge the pupil after breaking any posterior synechiae with the tip of the cannula. Introduce one hook from the paracentesis and the other through the wound. The two axes of the hooks will initially be parallel to each other, and one will push the pupil away while the other will pull it toward the surgeon. Do that until the pupil is close to the angle, and maintain this position for a few seconds. Then, cross the hooks in the anterior chamber, and do the same in the perpendicular plane. Occasionally, the borders of the iris will bleed, but this is usually

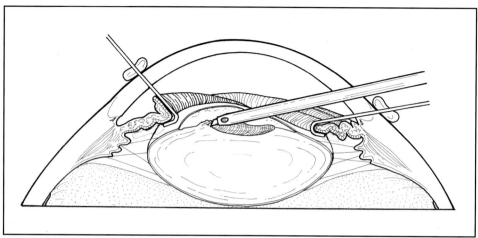

Figure 12-1 (Pearl 49). Iris hooks should be introduced parallel to the iris in the quadrants adjacent to the incision site to prevent upward iris tenting and contact with the surgical instruments. The hooks can be introduced more perpendicular to the iris plane in the other quadrants because this facilitates iris capture.

a self-limited problem. Next, remove the hooks, and fill the anterior chamber with viscoelastic material while starting in the center; this will push the pupil further in the periphery. The same maneuver can be repeated to attempt further dilation. If the pupil size is still inadequate, consideration should be given to using iris hooks.

Iris hooks are very helpful even when other strategies fail to achieve sufficient pupillary dilation. Having a set of iris hooks at a sufficient distance from the operating room may prevent falling in the trap of expediency to avoid waiting a few minutes to obtain the most adequate surgical tools. There are several types of hooks, and some are autoclavable, therefore reusable. Start by performing four small paracentesis incisions in a square fashion, taking into consideration the location of the phacoemulsification needle entry site and the side port. While performing the superior incisions, be sure that the paracentesis blade enters parallel to the pupil. This will prevent tenting of the iris and will facilitate entry of the phacoemulsification tip in the anterior chamber without engaging the iris (Figure 12-1). When making the inferior incisions, aim somewhat perpendicular to the plane of the iris (see Figure 12-1). This will make it much easier to introduce the hooks. After engaging the iris with the four hooks, start pulling on the pupil gradually until the size is adequate. Other commercially available devices help in pupillary dilation such as the Beehler pupil expander (Asico, Westmont, Ill), the Graether pupil expander (EagleVision (Memphis, Tenn), and the Perfect Pupil system (Becton-Dickenson, Waltham, Mass).

Iris hooks can also be used if the iris is damaged during phacoemulsification, becoming flaccid with an increased tendency to become aspirated. Occasionally, an iris fibril will float repeatedly into the phacoemulsification needle or the I/A cannula. Long Vannas scissors may be used to excise it. Sculpting away from the affected uvea should be attempted if possible. If this is not successful, then the use of a single iris retractor hook in that area will help keep the damaged tissue from being aspirated again.

Following lens extraction and IOL implantation, use Miostat (Alcon Surgical, Fort Worth, Tex) (carbachol 2%) to help constrict the pupil. Usually, the effect of Miostat is noticeable the next day. If the pupil size at the end of the procedure is large, the capsulorrhexis forceps may be helpful to pull on the iris and further constrict the pupil. Reach across the anterior chamber and pull the iris in toward the center. Repeat the same maneuver under the wound incision. Try to get the iris to cover the IOL because this will prevent iris/IOL capture. A Sinskey hook may be useful to break some superficial iris fibers in the desired quadrant, which will permit better pupillary constriction (Figures 12-2 and 12-3).

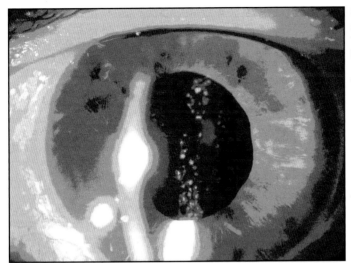

Figure 12-2 (Pearl 49). No attempt was made at constricting the pupil past dilation during phacoemulsification, causing patient glare and night vision problems. Note the iridectomy performed temporally due to iris prolapse during surgery.

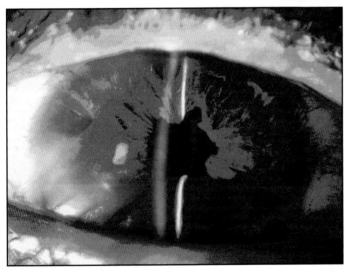

Figure 12-3 (Pearl 49). A glaucoma patient on chronic miotics and past multiple trabeculectomies underwent phacoemulsification with iris stretching with hooks. Carbachol 2% (Miostat) was placed at the end of surgery with resultant small pupil.

Always Remember...

Avoid tearing the anterior capsule as you are engaging the push-pull or the iris hooks.

Paradoxically, a small pupil may remain dilated after mechanical stretching. Patients should be informed of this possibility prior to surgery.

PEARL #50: THE HIDDEN CAPSULORRHEXIS

When the pupil size is 4 to 5 mm after dilation, the surgeon might want a larger size capsulorrhexis to safely proceed with cataract extraction. Observing the CCC leading edge is ordinarily valuable to prevent radial extension of the anterior capsular tear toward the periphery. It is possible to create a CCC larger than the pupil size by using the pupillary edge rather than the tear edge as a landmark. This can be performed by using the iris edge to guide the CCC incision (Figure 12-4). Clearly, this technique has a major limitation, which is the inability to salvage (and often detect) radial extension of the capsulorrhexis. Lastly, this maneuver may avoid iris manipulation but is also technically difficult to master.

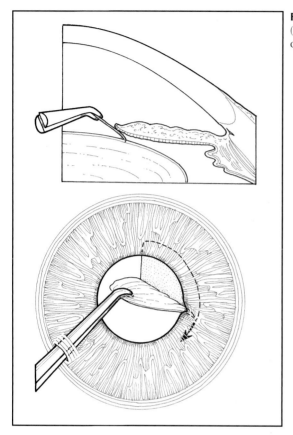

Figure 12-4 (Pearl 50). In pupils of moderate size (4 mm), the iris edge can be used as a guide to create a capsulorrhexis larger than the exposed capsule.

PEARL #51: THE FLOPPY IRIS SYNDROME

Iris prolapse may be due to an abnormality of the iris known as the "floppy iris syndrome" or due to intraoperative complications such as inadequate wound construction. The floppy iris syndrome has been attributed to PO intake (ie, oral intake) of Flomax (Boehringer Ingelheim, Ridgefield, Conn) prior to surgery and can be minimized by discontinuation of the drug for ≥2 weeks preoperatively; we have noted instances of the floppy iris syndrome 1 year after Flomax stoppage. At the time of surgery, decisive steps should be taken to avoid a disastrous cascade of events. A peaked pupil and decreased pupil size accompany iris prolapse. This will interfere with the capsulorrhexis, phacoemulsification, and the I/A steps. Repeated friction caused by the phacoemulsification tip may lead to iridodialysis and bleeding from the iris root. Postoperative iris atrophy, uveal incarceration, and cystoid macular edema might ensue.

Preoperatively, a few days of topical atropine administration has been suggested to minimize iris flaccidity. In addition, other intracameral preservative-free medications have been advocated to help with this condition. Paying special attention to the entry site into the anterior chamber may significantly minimize the incidence of iris prolapse during cataract surgery. Placing the keratome incision anterior to the corneal vascular arcade often prevents this complication. Several other surgical factors may contribute to iris prolapse including increased posterior vitreous pressure and a flaccid iris texture (in older individuals, in pseudoexfoliation syndrome, after stretching the pupil, and in some cases of high myopia).

Once iris prolapse occurs, the cause needs to be determined and the situation corrected prior to proceeding with surgery. Several strategies could be used if a posterior entry is determined to be the culprit. Introduce a cyclodialysis spatula through the paracentesis port, and gently sweep the iris from the root toward the center, while injecting sufficient but not excessive amounts of retentive viscoelastic material on top of the iris. Alternatively, insert a 3-mm lens sheath-glide made specifically for small-incision cataract surgery (Visitec [Becton Dickson, Franklin Lakes, NJ]). You may also trim a larger sheath-glide to the desired size. The glide will help you trap the iris underneath it. The phacoemulsification needle is introduced on top of the glide, and the case may proceed without further trauma to the iris. Another technique involves performing an iridectomy in the part of the iris that is prolapsing. This will allow anterior chamber fluid egress through the iridectomy and may relieve the uveal ballooning.

If these measures are successful, avoid multiple entries in the anterior chamber, whether with the phacoemulsification needle or the I/A cannula, to avoid additional uveal trauma (one can use bimanual I/A cannulas by creating another paracentesis and avoid going through the main incision). Similar measures may have to be taken at the time of IOL insertion. If the above strategies fail, it is preferable to close the incision and construct a more anterior entry site.

At the end of the procedure, special attention is needed to avoid uveal incarceration in the cataract wound. This may occur due to the flaccid iris resulting from earlier manipulation. In addition to miotic agents, a small amount of viscoelastic may be introduced from the paracentesis and injected on the iris plane below the wound to keep it separated from the corneal/scleral tissue. Tight sutures may be necessary to avoid subsequent pupil incarceration.

Always Remember...

Iris prolapse is not only due to an inappropriate incision. It may result from increased IOP secondary to malpositioned speculum, excessive viscoelastic agent, or suprachoroidal hemorrhage.

Concider discontinuation of Flomax prior to cataract surgery.

If the iris prolapse persists, suturing of the incision site and creating a new incision may be beneficial.

PEARL #52: TIPS FOR IRIS SUTURES

If the pupil remains too large even after the constricting measures described above, consideration should be given to placing iris sutures. This is especially important if the iris does not cover the IOL edge, which could potentially lead to visual aberrations. Spending a few minutes to place one or more iris sutures may save the patient (and the surgeon) significant aggravation, especially if a second procedure proves to be necessary.

10-0 prolene is best suited for iris suturing due to its durability. A CI-F4 needle is used if a McCannel-type technique is performed. The needle is passed through the cornea, in mid-iris (x2) then out through the cornea on the opposite side. Care should be taken to inflate the chamber to avoid operating on a soft globe. This will facilitate entry of the needle through the cornea. Creating paracentesis incisions through which the needle is introduced greatly facilitates this step. A Sinskey hook can then be introduced through the wound to bring out both ends of the sutures. These are then tied, and a Y-hook can be used to slide the knot into the chamber toward the iris before placing the locking suture (see Pearl #58).

Some cases of severe trauma may be left with significant iris fissure gaps despite suturing (Figure 12-5A). A cosmetic tinted contact lens may provide relief from glare symptoms (Figure 12-5B).

Always Remember...

Placing the suture bites in mid-iris will avoid "cheese-wiring" through the iris stroma.

Paracentesis incisions performed with the McCannel technique should be vertical to facilitate suture retrieval from the anterior chamber.

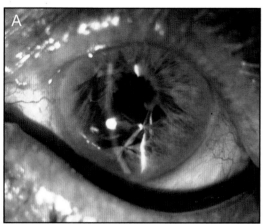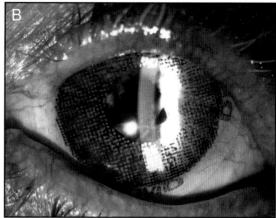

Figure 12-5 (Pearls 52). (A) Some cases of severe trauma may be left with significant iris fissure gaps despite suturing. (B) A cosmetic tinted contact lens may provide relief from glare symptoms.

BIBLIOGRAPHY

Chang DF, Campbell JR. Intraoperative floppy iris syndrome associated with tamsulosin. *J Cataract Refract Surg.* 2005; 31(4):664-673.

Chen V, Shochot Y, Blumenthal M. Anterior capsulotomy through a small pupil. *Am J Ophthalmol.* 1987;104(6):666-667.

Dinsmore SC. Modified stretch technique for small pupil phacoemulsification with topical anesthesia. *J Cataract Refract Surg.* 1996;22(1):27-30.

Faust KJ. Modified radial iridotomy for small pupil phacoemulsification. *J Cataract Refract Surg.* 1991;17(6):866-867.

Fine IH. Pupilloplasty for small pupil phacoemulsification. *J Cataract Refract Surg.* 1994;20(2):192-196.

Gimbel HV. Nucleofractis phacoemulsification through a small pupil. *Can J Ophthalmol.* 1992;27(3):115-119.

Graether JM. Graether pupil expander for managing the small pupil during surgery. *J Cataract Refract Surg.* 1996;22(5):530-535.

Mackool RJ. Small pupil enlargement during cataract extraction. A new method. *J Cataract Refract Surg.* 1992;18(5):523-526.

Masket S. Avoiding complications associated with iris retractor use in small pupil cataract extraction. *J Cataract Refract Surg.* 1996;22(2):168-171.

McCannel MA. A retrievable suture idea for anterior uveal problems. *Ophthalmic Surg.* 1976;7(2):98-103.

Miller KM, Keener GT Jr. Stretch pupilloplasty for small pupil phacoemulsification. *Am J Ophthalmol.* 1994;15;117(1):107-108.

Nelson DB, Donnenfeld ED. Small-pupil phacoemulsification and trabeculectomy. *Int Ophthalmol Clin.* 1994;34(2):131-144.

Pallin SL. Closed chamber iridoplasty. *Ophthalmic Surg.* 1981;12(3):213-214.

Yuguchi T, Oshika T, Sawaguchi S, Kaiya T. Pupillary functions after cataract surgery using flexible iris retractor in patients with small pupil. *Jpn J Ophthalmol.* 1999;43(1):20-24.

CHAPTER 13

TWO
PEARLS IN PHACOFLUIDICS AND BIMANUAL PHACOEMULSIFICATION

Tais Hitomi Wakamatsu, MD and Dimitri T. Azar, MD

PEARL #53: PHACOEMULSIFICATION FLUIDICS

Modern phacoemulsification techniques are less traumatic than earlier methods. Refinements in power modulation and control have led to reductions in the amount of ultrasonic energy delivered to the eyes. This considerably reduces turbulence in anterior chamber, which reduces the risk of injury to the corneal endothelium and the incision. If ultrasound (U/S) power is reduced, fragmentation ability must be increased; this is obtained by increasing contact between the nucleus and the U/S tip. But how is this obtained?

The fluidics aspect of all phacoemulsification machines is fundamentally a balance of fluid inflow and fluid outflow to maintain a constant intraocular volume and a stable and deep anterior chamber. The fluidic circuit is supplied via the silicone sleeve's irrigation ports by an elevated irrigating bottle that supplies both the fluidic volume and the pressure to maintain the chamber hydrodynamically (when the aspiration port is unoccluded and the pump is aspirating fluid and emulsate from the eye) and hydrostatically (when the pump is inactive, or when it is active with a complete occlusion of the aspiration port), respectively. Anterior chamber pressure is directly proportional to the height of the bottle.

The flow rate is the quantity of fluid that is aspirated in unit time (cubic centimeters per minute [cc/min]). Aspiration is important for mobilizing lens fragments and drawing them toward the aspiration orifice. The flow rate determines the speed at which the masses are drawn or removed. During the fragmentation phase, a higher flow rate will allow the U/S tip a greater capacity for attracting material. A high flow rate will equal U/S and vacuum values. However, very a fast flow rate can decrease your safety margin by quickly drawing in potentially unwanted materials (iris and capsule) as well as allowing less reaction time for reflux because of the corresponding rapid rise time. Therefore, greater control can be achieved by using more moderate flow rates and working in the area closer to the tip. When a fragment completely occludes the tip, the pump provides a vacuum of holding power measured in mm Hg, which grips the fragment to allow for further manipulation (eg, chopping). During the operation, the flow rate must be sufficient to mobilize and capture smaller fragments. Once this has happened, the vacuum must be able to keep the material held to the tip until it is fragmented and aspirated (during occlusion, the flow rate will decrease regardless of how fast the vacuum increases). After removal of the pieces that have been captured and that obstruct the tip, the vacuum returns to its previous values and the flow rate is reestablished. A pump with a low flow rate provides a greater safety margin even though it involves longer operating times. The ideal situation is to utilize a flow rate suitable for the needs of each operation.

If the irrigation is insufficient, however, shallowing of the chamber will occur. When prompt elevation of the bottle fails to increase the infusion, an air block, a venting problem, faulty tubing, or even an error in preparations is probably responsible. A wound of insufficient size might compress the collapsible sleeve that accompanies some systems. Kinking of this sleeve may also compromise infusion, resulting in chamber shallowing. In contrast to a tight incision, an incision that is too large allows fluid to escape. A subtler problem is a tendency for the surgeon to elevate the instrument, which causes the wound to gape and the chamber to empty. If too large an incision is made, placement of a single radial suture will often tighten the wound enough to inhibit egress of fluid. Alternatively, a new incision site may be selected.

Insufficient aspiration, like insufficient irrigation, may also occur because of an insufficient vacuum level, obstruction of the tube, obstruction of the tip and/or aspiration tube of the handle by part of the dense nuclear material or by the material that has not been completely fragmented, or because of wrong settings of vacuum or flow rate in the phaco machine.

If the flow of fluid is reduced or interrupted, the heat energy may be imparted to tissue in direct contact with the probe and, in particular, the corneoscleral wound site. The resulting damage may result in difficulty with wound leakage as well as damage to the adjacent corneal stroma and endothelium, fistula formation, and induction of high degrees of astigmatism. The main factor involved in the development of a "phacoburn" is a decrease in flow of irrigation and/or aspiration. It is important for surgeons to be aware of the fact that both clinical observation and experimental data indicate that a "phacoburn" develops over 1 to 3 seconds. Use of a precooled, balanced salt solution for irrigation has been suggested but is not currently generally employed. Verification of adequate irrigation flow before insertion of the phacoemulsification probe into the eye should always be performed. Once the probe has been inserted into the eyes and both irrigation and aspiration have been established, the deep chamber should be monitored to verify that irrigation and aspiration are well-sized solutions. Preferable techniques have been described as follows: a temporal approach is preferable; rigid, noncompressible sleeves have been developed as an alternative to soft silicone sleeves to decrease the risk of sleeve compression; placement of a groove on the phacoemulsification needle serves to maintain an irrigation channel despite sleeve collapse.

Always Remember...

In order to realize the full potential of a phaco machine, the surgeon must understand the logic behind setting the parameters of the bottle height, ultrasound power, vacuum, and flow.

PEARL #54: BIMANUAL PHACOEMULSIFICATION

Cataract surgery and phacoemulsification techniques have advanced dramatically over the past years. The development has been toward less traumatic surgery. Refinements in new techniques and instrumentations have offered a number of attractive benefits to both the surgeon and patient. The principal advantage is a smaller incision size, which decreases the amount of time injury, reduces the amount of postoperative pain and inflammation, and provides a more rapid refractive stabilization with less astigmatism induced by the procedure. The smaller incision also allows minimal restrictions on the patient's physical activities, even in the early postoperative period.

The notion of removing the crystalline lens through two microincisions is not new and has been attempted since the 1970s with varied success. With the development of the new phacoemulsification technology and power modulations, we can emulsify and fragment less material without generating significant thermal energy. Thus, the alternate method involves separating the irrigation from the ultrasonic aspirating tip and inserting each hand piece through separate incision ranging from the 1.2 to 1.5 mm in width. This bimanual microincision phaco (ie, microphaco) utilizes a bar ultrasonic needle (typically 20 Ga) without the use of the traditional surrounding silicone infusion sleeves, limiting the potential for thermal incision injury due to friction from the bare vibrating ultrasonic needle (eg, Bausch & Lomb Micro Flow [Rochester, NY], Alcon Hyperpulse [Fort Worth, Tex], AMO Whitestar).

Although currently no IOL will fit though a small stab incision, there are obvious advantages of lens extraction through two small incisions, including the ergonomic choice of switching instruments for more choices in angles of approach to anterior chamber contents with the aspiration port. Also, having irrigation once separate instrument allows more choices for directing the irrigating flow in order to purposely move material toward the aspiration port or, alternatively, to actively avoid problem areas such as weak zonules or a compromised capsule.

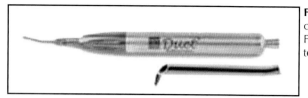

Figure 13-3 (Pearl 54). Duet bimanual irrigating chopper (top) and magnified view of the tip of the Fine irrigating vertical chopper (right). (Photos courtesy of MST MicroSurgical Technology.)

The major advantage of bimanual microincisions is an improvement in control of most endocapsular surgery steps. Because viscoelastic material does not leave the eye easily through these small incisions, the anterior chamber is more stable during capsulorrhexis construction and there is less likelihood for an errant capsulorrhexis to develop.

Surgical Techniques

Two clear corneal incisions are made by a 19- to 20-gauge keratome: one incision on the temporal limbus or superior temporal, as some surgeons prefer to do for the small phaco tip, and the other incision 60 to 90 degrees away for the side port. A 26-gauge needle on an ultra-small incision anterior capsule forceps is used to perform continuous curvilinear capsulorrhexis with a diameter of 5.0 mm after the hydrodissection is started. To prevent an abrupt rise in anterior chamber pressure, it is important to press the base of the hydrodissection needle firmly against the lower side of the incision so that excess fluid can leak out of the incision during the procedure. The infusion cannula is inserted through the side port; the sleeveless phaco tip is inserted through the temporal or superior temporal clear corneal incision; nucleofractis is carried out using the hook at the tip of the infusion cannula; and the nucleus is treated the same as in conventional phacoemulsification. The surgeon can perform bimanual phacoemulsification using an appropriate nucleofractis method such as divide and conquer, phaco chop, or quick drop (Figure 13-1). Infusion flow may not keep up with aspiration flow if aspiration is continued when there are no nuclear particles to be captured by the aspiration port on the phaco tip. Surgery can be performed more safely if aspiration is turned off when it is not needed. To improve the safety of this surgery, it is important to prevent the dispersion of nuclear fragments in the anterior chamber. Because nuclear fragments tend to disperse more readily with phacoemulsification and aspiration procedures than with other conventional techniques, it is best to set the ultrasound power as low as possible, reducing the extent of endothelial from the nucleus "kick." Care must also be taken when using the nucleofracts hook to handle nuclear fragments. In the emulsification of hard nuclei, considerable heat can be generated by the phaco tip, making it necessary to provide sufficient leakage of infusion solution through the incision to cool the tip and prevent thermal burn. In such cases, a 19-gauge microvitreoretinal (1.4 mm) is used to create the incision for the 20-gauge phaco tip. With relatively soft nuclei, the tip temperature can be reduced by turning down the ultrasound power and performing phaoemulsification and aspiration in pulse mode. Under these conditions, there is less need to cool the phaco tip by increasing the leakage of infusion solution through the incision. If the nucleus is soft, the initial corneal incision can be reduced even further using a 20-gauge microvitreoretinal keratome (1.2 mm) to make the incision for a 20-gauge phaco tip. This increases the stability of the anterior chamber during surgery and reduces injury to the corneal endothelium from the dispersion of nuclear fragments. The residual cortical fragments can be aspirated through an ultrasmall incision using a sleeveless infusion and aspiration tip or a 23-gauge side-port aspiration cannula (Figure 13-2). If the subincisional cortex is difficult to extract, the infusion and the aspiration cannula can be alternated between the two incisions to gain easier access to the subincisional capsule fornix. The IOL is inserted by an injector though a small incision enlarged between 2.5 and 3.2 mm.

Disadvantages

The disadvantages of bimanual phacoemulsification are real but easy to overcome. Maneuvering through 1.2-mm incisions can be awkward early in the learning curve. Capsulorrhexis construction

Figure 13-4 (Pearl 54). Magnified view of duet aspiration tip (left) and irrigation tip utilized for bimanual I/A (right). (Photo courtesy of MST MicroSurgical Technology.)

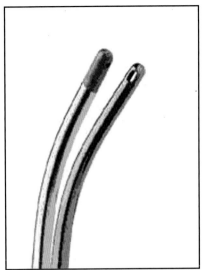

requires the use of a bent capsulotomy needle or specially fashioned forceps that have been designed to perform through these small incisions. Although more time is initially required, with experience, these maneuvers become routine. Also, additional equipment is necessary in the form of small-incision keratomes, rhexis forceps, irrigating choppers, and bimanual I/A hand pieces.

The greatest limitations of bimanual phaco lie in the fluidics and the current limitations in IOL technology that could be utilized through these microincisions. By nature of the size of these incisions, less fluid flows into the eye than occurs with coaxial techniques. Most current irrigating choppers integrate a 20-gauge lumen that limits fluid inflow. This can result in significant chamber instability when high vacuum levels are utilized and occlusion from nuclear material at the phaco tip is cleared. In the highest infusion designs, the chopping tip is attached peripherally to the irrigation needle so that the lumen can convey the maximum flow possible for a given gauge. Additionally or alternatively, surge can be limited with bimanual phaco by the use of various surge suppression devices (eg, small lumen phaco needles, small lumen aspiration lines, or the Staar "Cruise Control") or by augmenting inflow volume with an anterior chamber maintainer (as has been described by Michael Blumenthal, MD).

Always Remember…

Although coaxial phacoemulsification is an excellent procedure with low amounts of induced astigmatism, bimanual phacoemulsification offers the potential for truly astigmatic neutral incisions. In addition, these microincisions should behave similarly to a paracentesis incision with less likelihood for leakage and, theoretically, a lower incidence of endophthalmitis.

BIBLIOGRAPHY

Braga-Mele R, Liu E. Feasibility of sleeveless bimanual phacoemulsification with the Millennium microsurgical system. *J Cataract Refract Surg.* 2003;29(11):2199-2203.

Donnenfeld ED, Olson RJ, Solomon R, et al. Efficacy and wound-temperature gradient of whitestar phacoemulsification through a 1.2 mm incision. *J Cataract Refract Surg.* 2003;29(6):1049-1050.

Jaffe NS, Jaffe MS, Jaffe GF. *Cataract Surgery and Its Complications.* 6th ed. 1997:57-131.

Oki K. Measuring rectilinear flow within the anterior chamber in phacoemulsification procedures. *J Cataract Refract Surg.* 2004; 30(8):1759-1767.

Sakamoto T, Shiraki K, Inoue K, Yanagihara N, Ataka S, Kurita K. A simple, safe bimanual technique for subincisional cortex aspiration. *Ophthalmic Surg Lasers.* 2002;33(4):337-339.

Seibel BS. *Phacodynamics: Mastering the Tools and Techniques of Phacoemulsification Surgery.* 4th ed. Thorofare, NJ: SLACK Incorporated; 2005:2-51;156-172.

Sippel KC, Pineda R. Phacoemulsification and thermal wound injury. *Seminars in Ophthalmology.* 2002;17(3-4):102-109.

Soscia W, Howard JG, Olson RJ. Bimanual phacoemulsification through 2 stab incisions. A wound-temperature study. *J Cataract Refract Surg.* 2002;28(6):1039-1043.

Steinert RF. *Cataract Surgery: Technique, Complications, and Management.* 2nd ed. St. Louis, Mo: WB Saunders; 2004:61-77;469-486.

Tsuneoka H, Hayama A, Takahama M. Ultrasmall-incision bimanual phacoemulsification and ArySofSA30AL implantation through a 2.2 mm incision. *J Cataract Refract Surg.* 2003;29(6):1070-1076.

Tsuneoka H, Shiba T, Takahashi Y. Ultrasonic phacoemulsification using a 1.4 mm incision: clinical results. *J Cataract Refract Surg.* 2002;28(1):81-86.

Wilbrandt HR. Comparative analysis of the AMO Prestige, Alcon Legacy, and Storz Premiere phacoemulsification systems. *J Cataract Refract Surg.* 1997;23(5):766-780.

Fine IH, Hoffman RS, Packer M. Optimizing refractive lens exchange with bimanual microincision phacoemulsification. *J Cataract Refract Surg.* 2004;30(3):550-554.

CHAPTER 14

THREE
PEARLS IN AVOIDING PHACOEMULSIFICATION
CORNEAL BURNS

James J. Reidy, MD, FACS

In modern phacoemulsification surgery, ultrasonic power is produced within the hand piece by means of electrical stimulation of piezoelectric crystals contained within a transducer. Electrical stimulation of these crystals produces a high frequency vibration (28,000 to 60,000 Hz depending on the manufacturer) that is transmitted to the titanium needle, producing a longitudinal oscillation. The higher the amount of power applied, the greater the longitudinal stroke length of the needle. Emulsification of nuclear lens material within the fluid environment of the eye occurs by means of transient cavitation. Microbubbles are produced and release large amounts of energy in the form of shock waves immediately in front of the titanium needle, causing liquefaction of solid nuclear material.

Heat is produced within the fluid-filled confines of the eye during phacoemulsification by means of friction produced by the high-frequency oscillations of the phaco needle. Increased amounts of friction are produced when the vibrating phaco needle comes into contact with the irrigation sleeve. Heat production is moderated by inflow of fluid around the needle from the irrigation sleeve and outflow of fluid through the needle during aspiration. If fluid flow is inadequate, then temperatures high enough to produce tissue coagulation (60°C) may occur. Localized collagen shrinkage that results from excessive tissue temperatures can cause large amounts of astigmatism, wound leakage, and altered corneal wound healing. Thermal damage to the corneal endothelium in the area of the wound can result in localized corneal edema.

PEARL #55: PROPER HAND POSITIONING

Proper positioning of the patient and the surgeon can decrease the surgeon's tendency to elevate the hand piece during phacoemulsification. Elevation and torsion of the hand piece can result in localized wound compression, the location of which varies depending on the direction of the forces of compression. Compression of the phaco needle against the wound places it in direct contact with the irrigation sleeve, thereby interrupting fluid flow in this area and allowing focal heat production (Figure 14-1).

The operating table and the surgeon's chair should be adjusted so the surgeon's wrist is positioned below the patient's eye. In this position, the phaco hand piece will be parallel with the incision and results in less tendency to inadvertently elevate the hand piece, compressing it against the wound. When the wrist is elevated, the angle of tip insertion increases. A greater angle of insertion yields a greater amount of potential wound compression. Patients with deep orbits and prominent brows require a greater angle of insertion and attack to gain access to the anterior chamber when the incision is made superiorly. A temporal approach avoids the brow and improves access to the anterior chamber.

Always Remember…

Avoid elevating the phaco needle against the roof of the wound and lateral compression against the sides of the wound during application of phacoemulsification power.

A temporal approach is preferable in patients with deep orbits and prominent brows.

Use of an angled phaco tip decreases the need to elevate the hand piece during nuclear sculpting.

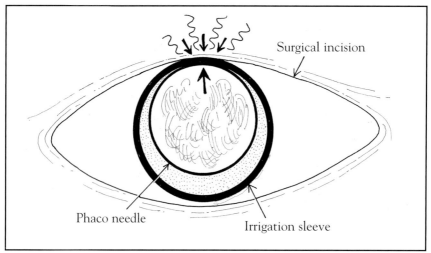

Figure 14-1 (Pearl 55). Compression of the phaco needle against the irrigation sleeve may generate significant focal heat and subsequent corneal burn.

Figure 14-2 (Pearl 55). A noncompressible internal Teflon sleeve around the phaco needle reduces the risk of compression-generated heat.

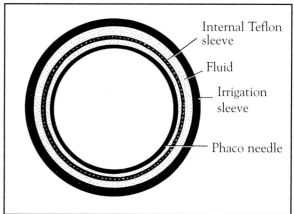

PEARL #56: APPROPRIATE IRRIGATION FLOW

The surgeon should ensure that there is adequate irrigation of fluid through the phaco tip prior to passing the phaco hand piece into the eye. Variable surgeon-controlled machine parameters, such as bottle height, aspiration flow rate, and vacuum, should be adequate to maintain a deep anterior chamber while allowing adequate inflow and outflow of fluid into and out of the eye. These parameters will vary based on surgical technique, the stage of the surgical procedure, density of the nucleus, and the specific machine being utilized.

The use of chilled irrigation solution (4°C) during phacoemulsification will increase the cooling capacity of the irrigation fluid. This temperature has no adverse affects on the corneal endothelium; in fact, corneas for transplantation are stored at this temperature.

Some phacoemulsification needles have been designed to minimize fluid inflow obstruction that occurs because of compression of the irrigation sleeve against the wound. Certain needles have a noncompressible internal Teflon sleeve (Figure 14-2), while others have external grooves distributed around the needle that permit fluid flow despite focal sleeve compression (Figure 14-3). Certain

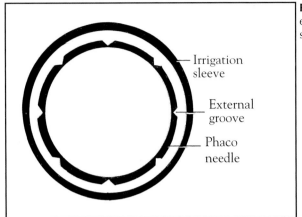

Figure 14-3 (Pearl 55). Externally grooved phacoemulsification needle permits fluid flow despite focal sleeve compression.

Irrigation sleeve

External groove

Phaco needle

irrigation sleeve designs employ spiral ridges that avoid fluid inflow obstruction. Although smaller diameter phacoemulsification needles may generate more heat, they have a smaller contact area when compressed against the wound, which maintains adequate cooling during such compression.

Always Remember...

Lowering the infusion flow rate to avoid excessively deep anterior chambers (eg, long axial length, postvitrectomy) may predispose to a corneal burn.

Sculpting the nucleus at zero vacuum settings may not provide adequate flow to ensure against corneal burns.

Consider a different phacoemulsification needle design and/or cooling the balanced salt solution if prolonged ultrasound is anticipated or if the problem of corneal burns recurs.

PEARL #57: DEBULK THE VISCOELASTIC IN THE ANTERIOR CHAMBER AND MINIMIZE THE USE OF ULTRASOUND POWER

Viscoelastic material that is placed into the anterior chamber prior to capsulotomy has the potential to temporarily occlude the phacoemulsification tip, especially if a highly retentive agent is used. This can be avoided if the viscoelastic is debulked with aspiration prior to initiation of phacoemulsification. This can be performed at the time when the anterior cortex is removed in the region of the capsulotomy.

Dense nuclei typically require somewhat greater phaco power to emulsify, which in turn, generates more heat. During nuclear sculpting, the least amount of ultrasound power that results in emulsification should be used. Shallow strokes should be employed to gradually shave down the nucleus and create a trough. Phacoemulsification should be interrupted on the backstroke.

Various techniques to break the nucleus into smaller pieces that are more amenable to removal with high aspiration will minimize the use of phaco power. Utilization of pulse or burst phacoemulsification modes during quadrant removal decreases the total amount of phaco time and, therefore, decreases heat production.

When the phaco needle becomes completely occluded with lens material, outflow through the lumen of the needle temporally ceases and heat production increases. In this situation, the surgeon should employ a higher level of aspiration combined with brief pulses (one second or less) of phacoemulsification power, which is achieved using the foot pedal or by switching the phaco mode to pulse or burst.

Always Remember...

Avoid overfilling the anterior chamber with viscoelastic material, especially if it has highly retentive properties.

Minimize the application of continuous phaco power to avoid excessive heat generation.

The use of pulse or burst modes for quadrant removal will decrease overall phaco time and lower the temperature generated by the phaco needle.

BIBLIOGRAPHY

Bissen-Miyajima H, Shimmura S, Tsubota K. Thermal effect on corneal incision with different phacoemulsification ultrasonic tips. *J Cataract Refract Surg.* 1999;25:60-64.

Davis PL. Phaco transducers: basic principles and corneal thermal injuries. *Eur J Implant Refract Surg.* 1993;5:109-112.

Mackool RJ. Preventing incision burn during phacoemulsification. *J Cataract Refract Surg.* 1994;20(3):367-368.

Majid MM, Sharma MK, Harding SP. Corneoscleral burn during phacoemulsification surgery. *J Cataract Refract Surg.* 1998;24:1413-1415.

FIVE PEARLS
IN THE MANAGEMENT OF CRYSTALLINE AND
ARTIFICIAL INTRAOCULAR LENS DISLOCATION

Ammar N. Safar, MD; Natalie A. Afshari, MD; and Alexandre Assi, Bsc, MBBS, FRCOphth

Dislocated crystalline or artificial IOLs may lead to temporary or permanent visual impairment. Zonular dialysis (eg, Marfan's syndrome and ocular trauma) or capsular bag compromise during cataract extraction may result in intraoperative crystalline lens dislocation with vitreous loss, retained nuclear fragments, and the need for further vitreoretinal surgery. Malpositioned artificial IOLs may also occur in situations of compromised capsular or zonular integrity during cataract extraction. This can lead to significant visual aberrations (eg, glare and diplopia) and loss of BCVA. This chapter will describe several techniques designed to successfully salvage IOL dislocation and to reposition displaced IOLs.

PEARL #58: POSTERIOR-ASSISTED LEVITATION

Preoperative scrutiny of the lenticular stability is essential for adequate planning and successful outcomes of cataract extraction in situations where zonular weakness may be present. Patients at risk include those with pseudoexfoliation, ectopia lentis syndromes (Marfan, Weill-Marchesani), and ocular trauma. Vitreous in the anterior chamber, phacodonesis, iridodonesis, and lens decentration (Figure 15-1) are strong indicators of significant zonular weakness. The remaining zonular support may falter at any point during cataract surgery, leading to lenticular dislocation into the vitreous chamber. Patients with normal preoperative zonular status may also encounter situations where the entire lens or lens fragments may tilt into the anterior vitreous, threatening to plunge toward the posterior pole. This may be due to intraoperative zonular dehiscence or to a large posterior capsular break.

Floating the tilted lens fragments on a cushion of viscoelastic material is not always successful. Dr. Charles Kelman described the technique of posterior-assisted levitation (PAL), which may be beneficial in cases of impending and early nuclear subluxation. However, this surgical technique is relatively invasive and may be associated with serious potential complications. The goal of the PAL maneuver is to elevate a falling nuclear fragment in order to permit either anterior chamber emulsification or manual extraction. The phacoemulsification tip is maintained in the eye with continuous irrigation to prevent the collapse of the globe. Alternatively, a 23-gauge butterfly needle may be introduced at the limbus as an anterior chamber maintainer. The infusion rate is decreased in order to prevent vitreous hydration and expansion of the capsular rent. A 23-gauge needle is then introduced through the pars plana 3 to 3.5 mm from the surgical limbus directly posterior to the remaining nuclear quadrant (Figure 15-2A). The needle should penetrate the eye oriented toward the optic nerve direction for 1.5 to 2 mm, then be reoriented and advanced horizontally until seen through the pupil. It is important to visualize the tip of the needle to ensure complete penetration of the ocular wall. The needle is then withdrawn until the tip is placed immediately below the nuclear quadrant. It is then used to impale or push the nuclear fragment upward into the pupillary plane. The prolapsed lens fragment is then removed through anterior chamber phacoemulsification or by enlarging the wound and expressing the fragment out of the eye. The needle is withdrawn and anterior vitrectomy and appropriate lens placement is carried out as indicated. Alternatively, a thorough vitrectomy may be performed through the pars plana if the surgeon feels comfortable with the technique. In situations where the needle provides sufficient support, a vitrectomy tip is introduced through another pars plana port, and the vitrectomy is performed prior to fragment elevation to minimize vitreous traction (Figure 15-2B). In cases where the whole lens dislocates, a

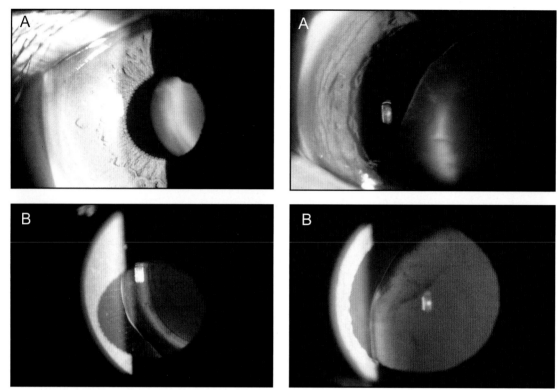

Figure 15-1 (Pearl 58). (A) Dislocated crystalline lenses secondary to traumatic damage to the zonules. (B) Retroillumination allows better examination of the zonular status.

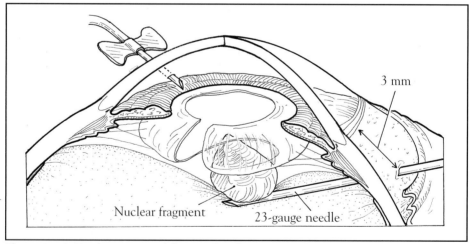

Figure 15-2A (Pearl 58). PAL. A falling nuclear fragment may be rescued and elevated into the anterior chamber using a needle introduced through the pars plana.

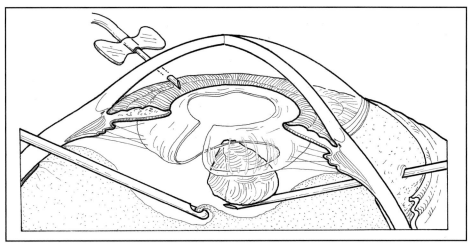

Figure 15-2B (Pearl 58). A 23-gauge butterfly cannula (connected to the balanced salt solution bottle) can be used as an anterior chamber maintainer. Simultaneous vitrectomy can minimize the risks of vitreous traction, especially in younger patients.

pupillary constricting agent can be injected after prolapsing the lens to trap it in the anterior chamber and facilitate its removal. Small nuclear fragments are difficult to manipulate with the needle and may not be as easily elevated into the anterior chamber.

Although PAL may be helpful in certain situations, the surgeon should be aware of its associated potential complications. These include injury to the ciliary body and bleeding as well as vitreous traction with possible retinal tears and detachment. In younger patients, pulling on the formed vitreous may predispose to retinal breaks. When faced with a falling lens, many surgeons believe that the safest course of action is to perform a thorough anterior vitrectomy and refer the patient to a vitreoretinal specialist for a pars plana lensectomy.

Always Remember...

Horizontal penetration of the eye may injure the ciliary body and result in hyphema or vitreous hemorrhage.

Complicated cataract surgery with vitreous loss increases the rate of postoperative complications. Dilated fundus examination with scleral depression is advisable in the early postoperative period.

PEARL #59: THE SHEATH GLIDE MANEUVER

The sheath glide, normally used during implantation of anterior chamber IOLs, can be useful to salvage a dislocated nuclear fragment following posterior capsular break during phacoemulsification. The glide is trimmed to fit the size of the clear corneal or scleral tunnel incision. Forceps are used to grasp the sheath and introduce it intraocularly. The sheath is advanced through the dilated pupil and positioned underneath the nuclear fragment to support it (Figure 15-3). In this position, the sheath glide also serves as a mechanical barrier in the face of any protruding vitreous. The phacoemulsification needle is then introduced through the incision anterior to the glide, and the fragment is removed. In cases where anterior vitreous protrusion is noted, vitrectomy should always be performed prior to nuclear manipulation.

Always Remember...

The sheath glide maneuver is most helpful when the inferior capsular bag is intact, such as in cases of subincisional posterior capsular defects.

Appropriate trimming of the sheath glide to fit the incision size is necessary for success of this maneuver.

Figure 15-3 (Pearl 59). A sheath glide can be used to prevent the dislocation of nuclear fragments into the vitreous in cases of a large posterior capsular break. The phacoemulsification needle can be introduced above the glide through the same incision.

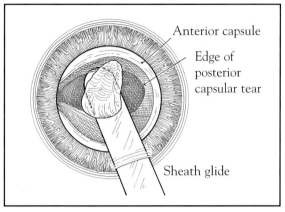

Anterior capsule

Edge of posterior capsular tear

Sheath glide

Pearl #60: McCannel Sutures for Dislocated Intraocular Lenses

The McCannel suturing technique is a useful procedure for repairing iris lacerations and repositioning dislocated IOLs. Several modifications have been described to enhance the safety of the procedure in managing dislocated or subluxed IOLs.

An adequate anterior vitrectomy is performed to disentangle the dislocated IOL from the surrounding vitreous. An intraocular forceps is then used to grasp the optic of the dislocated IOL and bring it forward into the anterior chamber. A pupil-constricting agent (eg, Miochol [CIBA Vision Corp, Atlanta, Ga]) is injected while the forceps continue to hold the IOL. When the pupil decreases in size to about 4 mm, the optic is prolapsed into the anterior chamber while the haptics are left in the ciliary sulcus (Figure 15-4A). Viscoelastic material is then layered over the iris, allowing adequate visualization of the orientation of both haptics of the incarcerated lens (Figures 15-4A and 15-4B). If needed, a Sinskey hook is used to orient the haptics in the desired meridian. 10-0 polypropylene on an STC-6 or CIF-4 needle (Ethicon, Somerville, NJ) is passed through the peripheral cornea into the anterior chamber, through the iris under the haptic, and out through the peripheral cornea. Limbal paracentesis usually facilitates the needle entry and exit through the cornea. Some surgeons may elect to leave the needle in place extending from its entry to its exit sites in the peripheral cornea with the iris and IOL haptic engaged with the needle (see Figure 15-4B). This will permit safe anchoring of the IOL while the other haptic is sutured to the iris.

A similar maneuver is used to suture the opposite haptic. The needle is pulled through, leaving the 10-0 prolene suture around the haptic. The needle is cut away, and both ends of the suture are captured with a Sinskey hook and pulled through a paracentesis created above the intended location of the suture knot (Figure 15-4C). The latter is created by starting the tying outside the eye and sliding the knot toward the iris using a Y-hook (Figure 15-4D) (see Chapter 12 for additional comments on iris sutures). The first needle is now pulled, and the prolene suture is tied to the haptic in the same manner. The optic is pushed back into the ciliary sulcus using a Sinskey hook or similar instrument.

Always Remember...

The IOL should be completely free from any vitreous attachment before attempting pupillary capture of the optic.

Sunset syndrome is less likely to occur if the haptics of the IOL are placed in the horizontal position.

Pearl #61: Double-Knot Transscleral Suture Fixation Technique for Sunset and Sunrise Syndromes

The terms sunset and sunrise syndromes have been coined to describe inferiorly and superiorly displaced lens optics, respectively. Figures 15-5A and 15-5B show examples of an inferiorly displaced IOL

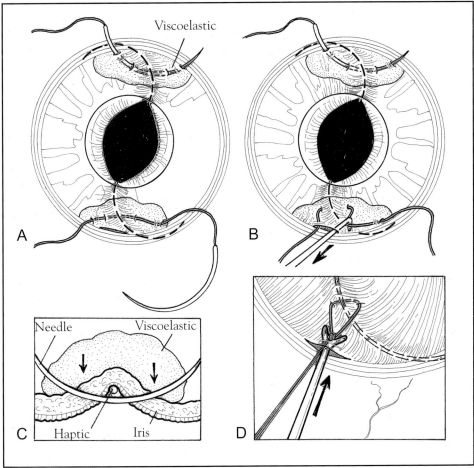

Figure 15-4 (Pearl 60). McCannel iris suture technique in IOL repositioning. (A, B, C) Viscoelastic material is injected on top of the iris to outline the location of the haptics after prolapsing the IOL optic into the anterior chamber. A CIF-4 needle is used to anchor the IOL haptic, while a McCannel suture is placed at the other haptic. (C) A Sinskey hook is used to retrieve the suture through a central paracentesis. (D) A Y-hook is used to slide the knot into the anterior chamber toward the iris-haptic.

(sunset syndrome) in both eyes of the same patient. Figure 15-5C shows an example of a superiorly displaced IOL (sunrise syndrome). This pearl describes a simplified technique by Azar et al to reposition displaced posterior chamber IOLs secondary to partial loss of zonule and posterior capsule support. This technique reduces intraocular manipulations and does not require special microsurgical tools.

An inferonasal displacement of the IOL with the superior haptic visible in the pupil will be used as an example (Figure 15-6A). A scleral flap is first created in the inferonasal quadrant. A paracentesis site is made superonasally. Through the flap, a straight needle is passed with a 10-0 prolene suture through the islet in the superior haptic (or anterior to the haptic if no islet is present), anterior to the iris, and then out of the eye through the paracentesis with the help of a 30-gauge needle serving as an exit guide wire (Figure 15-6B). A second needle is entered through the scleral flap and passed posterior to the haptic, exiting similarly at the paracentesis site (see Figure 15-6B). The two ends of the prolene suture are tied extraocularly (Figure 15-6C). Now, the superior haptic is connected by the prolene loop to the inferior flap. With the assistance of an intraocular forceps and a Sinskey hook, the IOL is brought up to the anterior chamber and rotated clockwise to bring the suture-looped haptic in line with the scleral flap and to bring the once-inferior haptic superiorly in line with the intact zonular support area

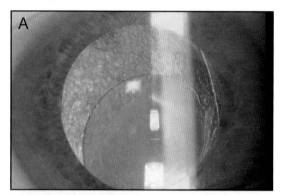

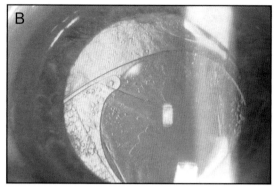

Figure 15-5 (Pearl 61). (A) Sunset syndrome: inferiorly displaced IOLs (right eye). (B) Sunset syndrome: inferiorly displaced IOLs in the left eye of the same patient. (C) Sunrise syndrome: superiorly displaced IOL.

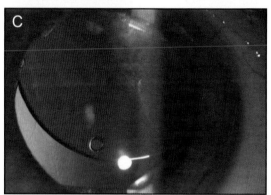

Figure 15-6 (Pearl 61). Double-knot transscleral suture fixation technique for displaced IOLs. (Reprinted with permission from Elsevier Science: Azar DT, Wiley WF. Double-knot transscleral suture fixation technique for displaced intraocular lenses. *Am J Ophthalmology.* 1999;128(5):645.)

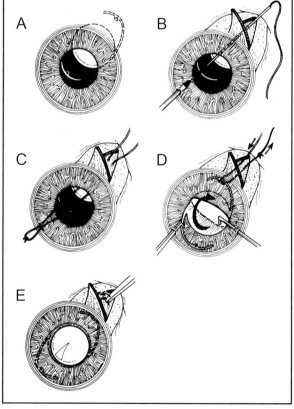

(Figure 15-6D). The IOL is replaced into the posterior chamber, and the suture is pulled to position the optic properly then tied to the sclera to tether the haptic in place. The first knot is discarded, while the second knot is trimmed and internalized with tying forceps (Figure 15-6E). The IOL is now well positioned and stable.

A modification to this surgical approach is to perform the flap in the superotemporal quadrant and pass the sutures in the manner described above to tether the superior haptic. This approach, however, does not add to inferior support of the IOL and may interfere with the intact superior posterior capsular support.

Always Remember…

Coverage of a scleral fixated IOL knot with a thick scleral flap will minimize the risk of suture exposure.

PEARL #62: DOUBLE-KNOT TECHNIQUE FOR IRIS FIXATION OF DECENTERED, DISLOCATED, OR SUBLUXATED SILICONE PLATE HAPTIC INTRAOCULAR LENSES

Silicone plate IOLs are more difficult to manipulate within the eye during IOL fixation than other lenses because they lack the easily grasped open-loop haptics. The one-piece silicone plate IOLs have a diameter of only 10.5 mm compared to the 14.0 mm diameter of foldable silicone haptic IOLs. As a result, a plate lens is more likely to decenter inferiorly. Decentered IOLs can be either repositioned or replaced by another lens. Azar et al have described an innovative repositioning technique to prevent the creation of large wounds needed for IOL explantation (Figure 15-7). This technique can be applied to reposition decentered, dislocated, or subluxated silicone plate haptic IOLs.

A limbal incision is made temporally (or nasally), and viscoelastic material is injected into the anterior chamber (Figure 15-7A). A curved needle with 10-0 prolene (CIF-4 needle) enters the anterior chamber through the incision and loops around the iris prior to its exit at the opposite end of the limbus (Figure 15-7B). An incision is then made superiorly, and suture ends are brought out of this incision with the help of a hook (Figure 15-7C). A hook is also passed through the temporal wound posterior to the iris to grasp the loop posterior to the iris and pull it out through the temporal incision (Figure 15-7D). Forceps are used to pull the plate lens through the pupil. A straight needle with 10-0 prolene suture enters the eye through the temporal incision and is passed though the eyelet of the IOL. This needle exits through the opposite limbus and then is cut (Figure 15-7E). A hook is passed through the temporal incision, and the end of the eyelet suture is brought out temporally (Figure 15-7F). At this point, two loops of suture (one attached to the IOL and the other passing through the iris) exit through the temporal incision (Figure 15-7G). The IOL is then rotated temporally, and the two loops are tied together near the eyelet of the IOL (Figure 15-7H). The superior suture is then gently pulled so that the IOL slips back under the pupil and is repositioned (Figure 15-7I).

Always Remember…

Iris fixation of a decentered silicone plate haptic lens requires minimal intraocular manipulation and avoids the need for IOL explantation and reimplantation.

BIBLIOGRAPHY

Alpar JJ. The use of Healon in McCannel suturing procedures. *Trans Ophthalmol Soc UK.* 1985;104(Pt 5):558-562.

Azar DT, Clamen LM. Iris fixation of a decentered silicone plate haptic intraocular lens. *Arch Ophthalmol.* 1998;116:821-823.

Azar DT, Wiley WF. Double-knot transscleral suture fixation technique for displaced intraocular lenses. *Am J Ophthalmol.* 1999;128(5):644-646.

Cionni RJ, Osher RH. Management of profound zonular dialysis or weakness with a new endocapsular ring designed for scleral fixation. *J Cataract Refract Surg.* 1998;24(10):1299-1306.

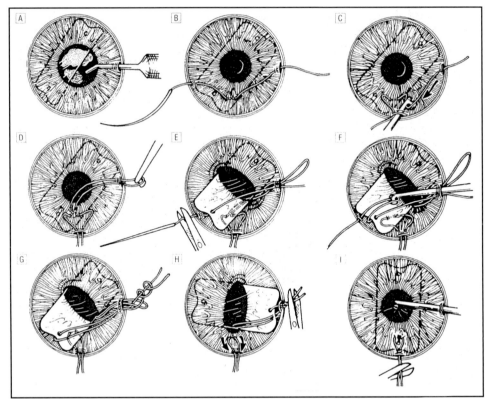

Figure 15-7 (Pearl 62). Double-knot technique for iris fixation of a decentered silicone plate haptic IOL. (Reprinted with permission from the American Medical Association. Iris fixation of decentered silicone plate haptic intraocular lens: double knot technique. *Arch Ophthalmol.* 1998;116:822.)

Clayman HM, Jaffe NS, Galin MA. *Intraocular Lens Implantation: Techniques and Complication.* St. Louis, Mo: CV Mosby; 1983.

Kelman C. Posterior capsular rupture: PAL technique. *Video J Cataract Refract Surg.* 1996;12:2.

McCannel MA. A retrievable suture idea for anterior uveal problems. *Ophthalmic Surg.* 1976;7(2):98-103.

Pallin SL. Closed chamber iridoplasty. *Ophthalmic Surg.* 1981;12(3):213-214.

Stark WJ, Michels RG, Bruner WE. Management of posteriorly dislocated intraocular lenses. *Ophthalmic Surg.* 1980;11(8):495-497.

CHAPTER 16

EIGHT
PEARLS FOR CHALLENGING CASES IN
CATARACT EXTRACTION

Richard Mackool, MD

This chapter describes special surgical techniques that can be extremely valuable when certain relatively common intraoperative complications/problems are encountered during cataract surgery.

PEARL #63: CAPSULAR DYES

These are indicated whenever difficulty is encountered with visualization of the anterior capsule during capsulorrhexis. The difficulty may be caused by an abnormality of the lens (white anterior cortical opacities or mature cataract), the cornea (corneal opacification of any etiology), or even the vitreous (vitreous hemorrhage with absent red reflex).

Indocyanine green (ICG) and trypan blue have been demonstrated to be safe when used for the purpose of anterior capsule staining, but there are differences with regard to cost. Trypan blue is relatively inexpensive.

The technique for use of these agents is identical. First, the anterior chamber may be filled with air, must this is not mandatory. This is most thoroughly accomplished if the injection of air is performed through a small side-port incision, which is located in a relatively dependent position. For example, slight elevation of the patient's head with injection of air at the 6 o'clock limbal position will normally result in a greater volume of air retention in the chamber because gravity causes the air to rise to the more superior portion of the chamber while aqueous passively drains from the eye alongside the cannula (a 27-gauge stainless steel cannula is recommended). Next, the staining agent is injected directly onto the surface of the anterior chamber, where it is permitted to remain for 5 to 10 seconds. Viscoelastic is then injected into the anterior capsule, replacing the air, and the capsulotomy is performed in the usual fashion. Alternatively, the dye can be injected beneath a viscoelastic agent and then "painted" on the anterior capsule using the side of the cannula. Additional viscoelastic injection then removes the dye from the chamber.

Dye Preparation

ICG dye comes in a bottle containing 25 mg lyophilized ICG powder with a second bottle of single-use diluent. The addition of 4.5 cc of BSS and 0.5 cc of the diluent to the ICG results in a concentration of 0.5% and osmolarity of 270 milliosmol (mOsm). Trypan blue is supplied as a premixed sterile solution.

Always Remember…

Do not hesitate to stain the anterior capsule whenever any opacities of the lens, cornea, or vitreous cause reduced intraoperative visualization.

PEARL #64: THE RUNAWAY RHEXIS

Successful capsulorrhexis is obviously a critical part of the phacoemulsification procedure. Escape of the capsular tear into the zonular region can result in a serious cascade of complications, including tear

Figure 16-1 (Pearl 64). If the capsulorrhexis starts to divert to the periphery, a spatula or other instrument can be inserted through a side port incision to depress the center of the nucleus in the region where the anterior capsule has been removed. This maneuver eliminates pressure on the anterior capsule by the nucleus and makes it easier to redirect the tear.

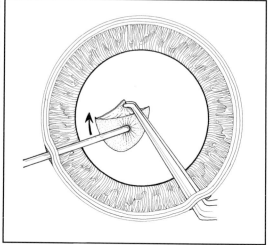

extension into the posterior capsule, vitreous loss or nucleus dislocation into the posterior segment, and postoperative IOL malpositioning.

Preoperative Warning Signs

Visible convexity of the anterior lens surface may encourage extension of the capsulorrhexis into the zonule (this convexity may also be a sign of zonular laxity). In general, it is safest to begin the capsulorrhexis centrally and to create a relatively small (3.5 to 5.0 mm) opening in this situation. If the rhexis proves to be too small for phacoemulsification, it can be enlarged (secondary capsulorrhexis).

Capsulorrhexis extension into the zonule is also more likely to occur in eyes having a shallow chamber or a tendency to become shallow during creation of the capsular tear. A high molecular weight viscoelastic can be helpful in such circumstances. Occasionally, the anterior chamber may be too shallow to permit either accurate capsulorrhexis or phacoemulsification. In these instances, removal of fluid from the posterior segment, preferably by a limited pars plana vitrectomy, is an excellent way to deepen the anterior chamber and is described in greater detail in Pearl 68.

At the first sign of "rhexis runaway," the following steps may be useful:

- Reinject viscoelastic to deepen the chamber.
- Insert a spatula or other instrument through a side port incision, and depress the center of the nucleus in the region where the anterior capsule has been removed (Figure 16-1). This maneuver eliminates pressure on the anterior capsule by the nucleus and makes it easier to redirect the tear.
- Grasp the anterior capsular flap approximately 1 to 2 mm from the advancing margin of the tear, and pull the capsule toward the center of the eye. If the tear can be redirected centrally, the capsulorrhexis can be completed as planned. However, if the tear extends into the zonular region, no further traction should be placed on the anterior capsular flap. The rhexis should be completed in the opposite direction (make a small cut in the capsulorrhexis margin in the opposite direction of the initial tear in order to initiate this). Thereafter, all chopping or nucleus cracking maneuvers should be performed at a location that is at least 90 degrees away from the capsulorrhexis extension.

Always Remember…

If the capsulorrhexis extends peripherally under the iris, a small cut in the capsulorrhexis margin in the opposite direction can be made to complete it from the opposite direction.

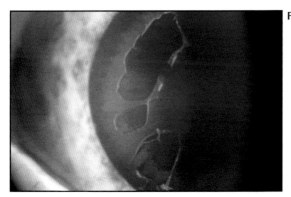

Figure 16-2 (Pearl 65). Pseudoexfoliation syndrome.

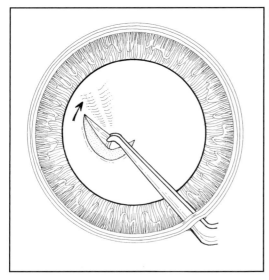

Figure 16-3 (Pearl 65). Watch for striae in the anterior capsule in advance of the tear as the capsulorrhexis is performed in patients with pseudoexfoliation syndrome. Such folds are evidence of decreased zonular traction, which would normally cause the capsule to remain taut.

PEARL #65: PSEUDOEXFOLIATION QUANDARY

In the majority of instances, eyes with pseudoexfoliation (Figure 16-2) behave normally during phacoemulsification. Unfortunately, this is not always the case, and in some patients, the zonule may be lax or even virtually absent. Therefore, it is recommended that each patient be advised of the presence of this condition and the impact that it may have upon the surgical procedure.

The intraoperative aspects of dealing with pseudoexfoliation can be divided into assessment of zonular status; steps to reduce zonular stress; and special techniques/instrumentation/devices.

Assessment of Zonular Status

Assuming that phacodonesis is not present preoperatively, evaluation of zonular status is first possible at the time of anterior capsule incision/capsulotomy. If a bent-tip needle is used to begin the capsulotomy, any shifting of the entire lens at this time is indicative of zonular weakness. Also, as the capsulorrhexis is performed, watch for striae in the anterior capsule in advance of the tear (Figure 16-3). Such folds are evidence of decreased zonular traction, which would normally cause the capsule to remain taut. Despite thorough hydrodissection, nuclear rotation may be difficult if the zonule does not maintain adequate tension on the equatorial lens capsule. The capsule may tend to rotate with the nucleus, and bimanual nucleus rotation (utilizing the phacoemulsification needle and a spatula or chopper or two other instruments such as Sinskey hooks or bent-tip needles) is an effective way to spin the nucleus while maintaining its location within the center of the lens capsule.

Surgical Steps to Avoid Zonular Stress

It is generally advisable to perform phacoemulsification with a lower infusion pressure and, therefore, lower aspiration flow rate and vacuum levels in these eyes. Lowering the infusion bottle by approximately 30 cm and using proportionately reduced flow and vacuum levels may cause the emulsification process to proceed more slowly, but this is recommended even if there is no evidence of zonular laxity. Bimanual rotation using the phaco tip and a second instrument, such as a phaco chopper or spatula, should be employed whenever possible.

If segmentation of the nucleus is to be done, it should obviously be accomplished as gently as possible. Deep sculpting will enable the nucleus to be cracked with less effort; if phaco chop is preferred, impaling the nucleus with the phaco tip permits it to be held in situ as it is chopped. If the zonule is extremely lax, it may be advisable to perform a capsulorrhexis that is large enough to permit elevation of all or part of the nucleus above the plane of the anterior capsule. Maintaining a dispersive viscoelastic anterior and posterior to the nucleus is highly recommended in such circumstances. Alternative measures are described in the following section (Special Techniques, Instrumentation, and Devices).

After nucleus removal, tangential stripping of lens cortex from the capsular fornices may prevent further zonular dehiscence. In extreme circumstances, it may be necessary to position the distal end of a second instrument, such as a blunt spatula, against the capsular fornix in order to create countertraction as the cortex is removed.

During IOL implantation, undue pressure against the capsular fornix with the haptic of the IOL should be avoided. In order to accomplish this, the distal haptic can be placed into the capsular sac in the usual fashion. A trailing haptic can then be dialed into the capsular sac while using a capsule retractor/lens guide to simultaneously retract the anterior capsule and the tip of the instrument functions as a guide for the trailing haptic. However, insertion of a single-piece acrylic lens is less stressful to the zonule because the soft haptics open slowly and gently within the capsule.

Special Techniques, Instrumentation, and Devices

Stabilization of the lens-zonule complex during cataract removal can be dramatically helpful. The instrumentation and devices that can be used to accomplish this are the endocapsular tension ring and retractors, which can be used to provide support to the lens capsule.

Endocapsular Tension Ring

When inserted into the capsular sac, an endocapsular ring provides a circumferential expansile force to the capsular equator. The capsule is therefore much less likely to be attracted to the phaco tip, and increased stability of the lens may be observed. However, these devices do not necessarily result in increased stabilization of the position of the cataract relative to other ocular structures, and they often entrap lens cortex between themselves and the lens capsule. Removal of the cortex can be extremely difficult, and in fact, traction can be transmitted to the capsule during such attempts; this can cause further structural damage to the zonule. Nonetheless, expansion of the capsular sac is often extremely desirable either during or after lens removal, and these devices do appear to reduce postoperative pseudophacodonesis and enhance implant centration.

Capsule Retraction Devices

Both iris retractors and specially designed lens capsule retractors have been used to stabilize the capsule and enclosed nucleus during phacoemulsification. Iris retractors, with which most surgeons are familiar, can be inserted and used to engage the margin of the capsulorrhexis. Multiple retractors are capable of providing fixation to the capsule; however, their relatively short length and single-plane design cause them to easily slip off the capsule during manipulation of the nucleus. In addition, iris retractors are short and do not extend into the capsular fornix; therefore, they do not offer support to this region.

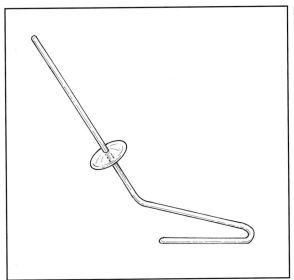

Figure 16-4 (Pearl 65). Anterior capsule retractor used in patients with pseudoexfoliation syndrome.

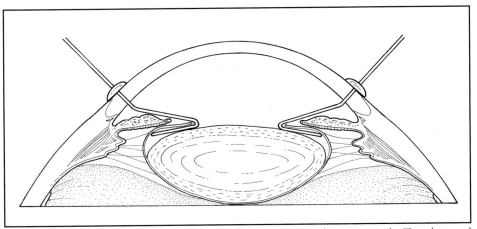

Figure 16-5 (Pearl 65). Six capsule retractors are placed at 45-degree intervals. The elongated return of the retractor extends into the capsular fornix and, therefore, functions to prevent attraction of the equatorial capsule to the phacoemulsification tip.

Because of these disadvantages, I designed retractors (Figure 16-4) that are specifically shaped for the purpose of retracting the anterior capsule. Although several minutes may be required to insert them, five or six retractors placed at 60- to 70-degree intervals provide superb and reliable support to the capsule and the enclosed nucleus. The elongated return of the retractor extends into the capsular fornix and, therefore, functions to prevent attraction of the equatorial capsule to the phacoemulsification tip (Figure 16-5). After nucleus and cortical removal are complete, an endocapsular ring can be inserted prior to removal of the retractors and insertion of an IOL.

Endocapsular Rings

Endocapsular rings can also be sutured to the sclera (Cionni design) (Figure 16-6). Such rings contain a small strut with a distal eyelet. Prior to insertion of the ring, a double-armed 10-0 prolene suture can be passed through the eyelet. After ring insertion, both needles are passed through the appropriate region of the ciliary sulcus and are tied to each other. It is preferable to accomplish this by inserting a 27-gauge disposable needle through the sclera, 1 mm posterior to the limbus, at the desired location.

Figure 16-6 (Pearl 65). An 11-year-old with Marfan syndrome and inferior lens disloca- tion. An endocapsular ring (Cionni design) was used to suture the capsular bag to the sclera. (Courtesy of Robert J. Cionni, MD, Cincinnati Eye Institute.)

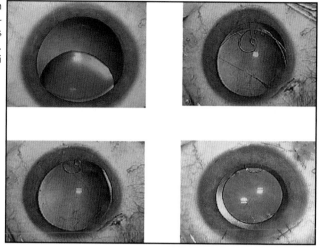

This needle is advanced through the region of the ciliary sulcus and into the anterior chamber anterior to the lens capsule. One of the two straight needles attached to the double-armed 10-0 prolene suture is then passed through the phaco incision (through which the endocapsular ring was inserted) and into the 27-gauge needle, which is then withdrawn from the eye. This "needle-pass" procedure is repeated: passing the straight needle at the other end of the double-armed suture through the sclera at a site that is approximately 0.5 to 1.0 mm from the first "needle-pass." The straight needles are then amputated, and the two ends of the suture are tied to each other in order to establish permanent positioning of the endocapsular ring and surrounding capsule. This technique is similar to those used for suturing posterior chamber lenses to the sclera, and other methods of accomplishing this can be successfully used.

Always Remember…

Pearl #66: The Shallow Anterior Chamber

Preoperative consideration should be given to the cause of chamber shallowing. Causes include a small anterior segment (usually but not always associated with a short axial length), a swollen lens with increased volume, and a lax zonule permitting the lens to shift forward. More rarely, a relative lens-block may be present in susceptible eyes. Such eyes are more likely to develop aqueous misdirection ("malignant" glaucoma) after cataract removal, especially if cataract removal is combined with filtration surgery.

If the zonule is extremely lax, the insertion of capsule retractors can stabilize the capsule and lens. Alternatively, a capsulorrhexis that is large enough to permit elevation of all or part of the nucleus above the plane of the anterior capsule could be created.

In patients with pseudoexfoliation syndrome, it is generally advisable to perform phacoemulsification with a lower infu- sion pressure and, therefore, lower aspiration flow rate and vacuum.

Regardless of etiology, a shallow anterior chamber can (1) make it extremely difficult to perform a capsulorrhexis that does not extend into the zonular region, (2) place the corneal endothelium at risk during phacoemulsification, and (3) increase the risk of intraoperative complications such as posterior capsule rupture and vitreous loss if an associated zonular laxity is present. Infusion misdirection, dis- cussed later in this chapter, is also more likely to occur in eyes with zonular laxity; if this develops, it is more often of clinical relevance because a small amount of misdirected fluid can place the posterior capsule in proximity to the phaco or I/A tip.

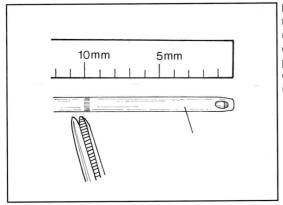

Figure 16-7 (Pearl 66). A mosquito clamp may be used to create superficial scratches on the surface of the vitrectomy tip by rotating the tip back and forth within the clamp. The tip can then be inserted through the pars plana and toward the geometric center of the vitreous cavity until the markings on the tip are located just external to the sclera.

The following recommendations are made in the order in which related problems may be encountered during the procedure:

- If adequate chamber depth cannot be obtained by viscoelastic injection, a partial pars plana vitrectomy should be performed in order to soften the eye and permit additional viscoelastic injection to create a deep chamber.
- No more than 0.25 cc of vitreous should be removed, during which time digital palpation of the globe should be used to verify IOP lowering.
- It is best to err initially on the side of too little vitreous removal, followed by gentle viscoelastic injection into the anterior chamber.
- If adequate chamber depth is not achieved, additional vitrectomy can be performed. In this manner, excessive removal of vitreous with extreme deepening of the anterior chamber can be avoided. However, if this should occur, removal of viscoelastic followed by gentle injection of BSS into the vitreous cavity through the pars plana opening can be performed in order to establish appropriate chamber depth.

Should the density of the cataract prohibit visualization of the vitrectomy tip behind the lens, the vitrectomy tip should be scored 10 mm from its distal end; grasping the tip with a serrated clamp can do this. The clamp is then used to create superficial scratches on the surface of the tip by rotating the tip back and forth within the clamp (Figure 16-7). The tip is then inserted through the pars plana and toward the geometric center of the vitreous cavity until the markings on the tip are located just external to the sclera. The vitrectomy can then be performed as described above.

These maneuvers require familiarity with standard methods and techniques for creating an incision through the pars plana. In brief, an inferotemporal incision site should be selected when possible, and the pars plana opening should be created with an appropriate-sized MVR blade. After completion of the vitrectomy and viscoelastic injection, the globe should remain slightly soft (ie, the IOP should never be greatly elevated by fluid injection while a pars plana incision remains open). Small amounts of vitreous may often be present within the sclerotomy, and they should be removed with the use of a weck sponge and small scissors. A 9-0 nylon suture should be used to tightly close the sclerotomy. The capsulorrhexis and phacoemulsification can then be performed in a routine manner. However, if zonular laxity is present, techniques used to deal with this situation may be required (see Pearl #67).

Should anterior chamber shallowing develop during the procedure (or for that matter, should it develop at any time during any phacoemulsification procedure), the possibility of infusion misdirection syndrome (IMS) or subchoroidal hemorrhage (SCH) must be considered. This situation is discussed in the next section.

Always Remember...

Always rule out SCH as a cause of unexplained anterior chamber shallowing.

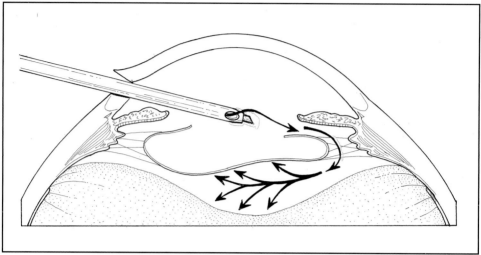

Figure 16-8 (Pearl 67). IMS.

PEARL #67: INFUSION MISDIRECTION SYNDROME

Because the zonule is porous, water molecules are able to pass through this structure at any time during phacoemulsification or I/A. If a significant volume of fluid does so, the condition is called IMS (Figure 16-8). The posterior capsule will be immediately displaced forward and may contact and/or be aspirated by the phaco or I/A tip. The following recommendations are made in the order in which related problems may occur during phacoemulsification:

- If persistent chamber shallowing is noted during phacoemulsification or I/A and the IOP is normal or elevated (this can be determined by placing the footpedal in position 1 and estimating IOP by digital palpation), then either IMS or SCH has occurred.
- If the chamber is shallow and the globe is soft, then there has been a failure to deliver adequate infusion to the eye, and appropriate investigation must be made to determine the cause (eg, kinked infusion line or empty infusion bottle).

The following steps should be taken in order to differentiate IMS from SCH:

- Inject viscoelastic slowly into the central region of the posterior chamber. If IMS is present, fluid may be displaced from the posterior segment, through the zonule, and into the anterior chamber. This would result in anterior chamber deepening. If this occurs, the problem can be presumed to be IMS.
- If the chamber does not deepen, indirect ophthalmoscopy is required in order to differentiate SCH from IMS. Do not hesitate to terminate the procedure and bring the patient to an examination area for indirect ophthalmoscopy or B-scan ultrasonography if the posterior segment cannot be visualized because of retained lens material, etc.
- If it is determined that choroidal detachment is not present, the patient has IMS, and this will usually resolve within 1 hour; the procedure can then be completed. A recurrence of IMS may be less likely if the infusion bottle is maintained at a low level and, appropriately, low flow rate and vacuum levels are employed.
- If SCH is diagnosed, the procedure should be terminated even if large amounts of nuclear or cortical material remain in the eye. In most cases, the procedure can be completed in approximately 2 weeks following consultation with a vitreoretinal specialist.

PEARL #68: TECHNIQUES FOR REATTACHMENT OF DESCEMET'S MEMBRANE

Detachment of Descemet's membrane (DM) may be more frequent, or at least more clinically recognizable, with the advent of clear corneal incisions. If the detachment is recognized during lens removal, the membrane must be protected from contact with any instruments as lens removal is completed. The injection of a dispersive viscoelastic in the region of attached DM will usually accomplish this. Care must be taken during the remaining portion of the procedure, especially during IOL insertion, to prevent further detachment, and this may require the creation of another incision 45 to 90 degrees away from the initial incision. At the conclusion of the cataract implant procedure, the anterior chamber should be filled as completely as possible with air.

In nearly every instance, the DM separation will originate from the surgical incision. However, tears in the membrane may radiate away from the incision, and it can be extremely difficult to determine their correct orientation. Therefore, it may be necessary and desirable to bring the patient to an examining area where slit lamp biomicroscopy can be performed to accurately map the detachment and location of membrane tears. It may also be necessary to apply topical glycerine to dehydrate the cornea for better visualization (unfortunately, the commercially available form of glycerine has recently been discontinued; it is available from some compounding pharmacies).

Reattachment Techniques

Injections of air, gas (SF6 or C3F8), and direct suturing have reportedly been successful in reattaching DM. If the detachment is relatively flat (not scrolled), reattachment is usually relatively simple and successful. An air injection, which may require repetition every 2 to 4 days for 1 to 2 weeks, will normally suffice. Although gas injection can provide significantly longer tamponade than air, there is greater endothelial toxicity with these chemicals. Viscoelastic injection should probably be reserved for those cases in which the membrane must be manipulated into anatomic alignment with the corresponding stroma (eg, DM scrolling) prior to reattachment. Using viscoelastic to accomplish this task creates the least trauma to the endothelium. However, the viscoelastic may insinuate itself between the membrane and the stroma and inhibit reattachment. If viscoelastic followed by air injection is performed, the patient will need to be monitored daily; air injection must be repeated in order to maintain alignment of the membrane for approximately 1 week.

Suturing of DM should probably be restricted to those unusual cases that are recalcitrant to the above techniques. Suturing is likely to cause significant endothelial trauma and should, therefore, be avoided whenever possible.

Patient Positioning

Following air or gas injection, the patient should be positioned in order to provide maximum contact of the air bubble with the torn region of DM. Unless the tear in DM extends into the inferior region of the cornea, this is usually relatively simple to accomplish. In the event of an inferior tear, however, positioning becomes more difficult (either Trendelenburg or seated position with head between legs is required).

With large and/or complex detachments, meticulous evaluation prior to repair is mandatory. This involves the creation of a detailed drawing indicating the areas, tears, and morphology of the detachment. Such a drawing will provide invaluable intraoperative guidance.

Always Remember…

Do not hesitate to stop the procedure if a DM detachment is suspected; perform a slit lamp examination using topical glycerine if necessary, and carefully plan the detachment repair.

PEARL #69: UPRIGHT PHACOEMULSIFICATION

Some patients are unable to assume the supine position normally required for cataract removal. If the patient is able to partially recline to approximately 45 degrees and has adequate neck extension, phacoemulsification may be possible (although this may require the surgeon to stand).

Figure 16-9 (Pearl 69). Upright phacoemulsification, the straddle position. The microscope must be appropriately positioned, and attention must be paid to obtaining adequate tilt of the microscope toward the surgeon so that the patient's brow does not obstruct visualization of the anterior segment.

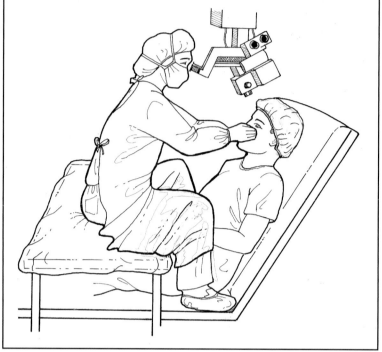

Rarely, the patient may need to maintain a near-sitting position, and this will require extraordinary measures if phacoemulsification is to be performed. These include the following.

- **Topical anesthesia**. Although not mandatory, this will permit the patient to assist the surgeon to obtain exposure of the inferior limbus by voluntary supraduction.

- **Unique positioning of the surgeon**. If it is possible for the patient to turn his or her head toward the right (for right eye surgery) or left (left eye surgery), the surgeon may sit beside the patient while performing phacoemulsification. This will require, however, that the surgeon rotate his or her torso toward the patient, and it may be somewhat difficult to maintain this position for the duration of the procedure. Alternatively, the surgeon may straddle the patient as described below.

- **The straddle position (Figure 16-9)**. In order to do this, a bench (a picnic bench works well for this) can be placed over the patient's legs. After the patient is prepped and the patient and the bench are draped, the surgeon mounts the bench, faces the patient, and places one leg on each side of the patient. Footstools are used to elevate the foot pedals for the phaco and microscope systems so that they are within reach of the surgeon. The microscope must be appropriately positioned, and attention must be paid to obtaining adequate tilt of the microscope toward the surgeon so that the patient's brow does not obstruct visualization of the anterior segment. It may be necessary to elevate the entire microscope by placing boards beneath its footings. An assistant may need to hold the lid speculum in position because the near vertical position of the patient's head encourages the speculum to "ride low."

The above procedure is clearly challenging, and it is strongly suggested that a dry run be made in the operating room prior to actually scheduling the procedure in order to troubleshoot any difficulties and verify that the patient, microscope, and equipment can be appropriately positioned. Lastly, remember that the ability to deliver infusion fluid to the eye is dependent on the distance between the eye and the drip chamber of the infusion bottle. Therefore, the infusion bottle will have to be markedly elevated from its usual position; an IV pole may be required, and ceiling height must be adequate for this. Alternatively, a nongravity (gas-pressurized) infusion system, if available, could be employed.

PEARL #70: INTRAOCULAR LENS POWER CALCULATION AFTER LASIK

The measurement of corneal power after laser vision correction (LASIK, PRK, LASEK) is well known to be problematic. A number of methods such as the clinical history, contact lens and over-refraction, and other techniques that estimate corneal power have been reported. These have problems: they estimate corneal power and the hard contact lens and over-refraction method relies on refraction in an eye with suboptimal acuity. I concieved the following method to eliminate these issues.

Aphakic Refraction Technique

The cataract is removed, temporarily rendering the patient aphakic. An aphakic refraction is performed shortly after cataract extraction (usually in about 20 to 30 minutes), and the IOL power is calculated based upon the spherical equivalent of that refraction. The patient then returns to the operating room for IOL implantation. The following should be noted:

- It is not necessary to perform the aphakic refraction and secondary IOL insertion on the same day as cataract removal. They may be done anytime within 2 to 3 weeks (adherence of the anterior and posterior capsules can be significant after that time, and IOL insertion into the capsular sac may therefore be difficult).

- If the aphakic refraction is performed on the same day, the cornea should be lubricated immediately after cataract removal and again just prior to performing the refraction. IOP should be at physiological levels at the time of the refraction.

I use the following nomogram for IOL power calculation. For an IOL placed within the capsular sac with an A-constant of 118.84, multiply the aphakic refraction by a conversion factor of 1.75 in order to obtain the dioptric power of the IOL if the spherical equivalent aphakic refraction is greater than +8.00. The conversion factor is 1.70 if the aphakic refraction is between +2.00 and +8.00, and the factor is 1.2 if the aphakic refraction is less than +2.00 (or myopic). Note that most aphakic refractions in these eyes will have a spherical equivalent of +8.00 or greater because they were likely made emmetropic or near emmetropic by the previous LASIK procedure. The refraction should be performed at a vertex distance of 12 mm, or corrected for it.

Lastly, it should be noted that this technique may be used for other situations, such as posterior staphyloma, that cause difficulty in measuring axial length and therefore IOL power determination.

BIBLIOGRAPHY

Aranberri J. Intraocular lens power calculation after corneal refractive surgery. Double-k method. *J Cataract Refract Surg.* 2003;29:2063-2068.

Cionni RJ, Osher RH. Management of profound zonular dialysis or weakness with a new endocapsular ring designed for scleral fixation. *J Cataract Refract Surg.* 1998;24(10):1299-1306.

Dietlein TS, Jacobi PC, Konen W, Krieglstein GK. Complications of endocapsular tension ring implantation in a child with Marfan's syndrome. *J Cataract Refract Surg.* 2000;26(6):937-940.

Drolsum L, Haaskjold E, Sandvig K. Phacoemulsification in eyes with pseudoexfoliation. *J Cataract Refract Surg.* 1998;24(6):787-792.

Faschinger CW, Eckhardt M. Complete capsulorrhexis opening occlusion despite capsular tension ring implantation. *J Cataract Refract Surg.* 1999;25(7):1013-1015.

Fine IH, Hoffman RS. Phacoemulsification in the presence of pseudoexfoliation: challenges and options. *J Cataract Refract Surg.* 1997;23(2):160-165.

Gimbel HV, Neuhann T. Development, advantages, and methods of the continuous circular capsulorrhexis technique. *J Cataract Refract Surg.* 1990;16(1):31-37.

Hoffer KJ. Intraocular lens power calculation for eyes after refractive keratotomy. *J Refract Surg.* 1995;11:490-493.

Holladay JT. IOL calculations following radial keratotomy surgery. *Refract Corneal Surg.* 1989;5:36A.

Kuchle M, Viestenz A, Martus P, et al. Anterior chamber depth and complications during cataract surgery in eyes with pseudoexfoliation syndrome. *Am J Ophthalmol.* 2000;129(3):281-285.

Lee V, Bloom P. Microhook capsule stabilization for phacoemulsification in eyes with pseudoexfoliation syndrome-induced lens instability. *J Cataract Refract Surg.* 1999;25(12):1567-1570.

Mackool RJ, Sirota M. Infusion misdirection syndrome. *J Cataract Refract Surg.* 1993;19(5):671-672.

Odenthal MT, Eggink CA, Melles G, et al. Intraocular lens power calculation for cataract surgery after photorefractive keratectomy. *Arch Ophthalmol.* 2003;121:1071.

Ridley F. Development in contact lens theory. *Trans Ophthalmol Soc UK.* 1948;68:385-401.

Soper J. Contact lens fitting by retinoscopy. In: Soper J, ed. *Contact Lenses: Advances in Design Fitting, Applications.* New York, NY: Stratton Intercontinent Medical Book Corp; 1974:99-108.

CHAPTER 17

FIVE
PEARLS IN LIMBAL STEM CELL
TRANSPLANTATION

Kimberly C. Sippel, MD and C. Stephen Foster, MD, FACS

PEARL #71: CORRECTLY IDENTIFY LIMBAL STEM CELL DEFICIENCY

The limbal epithelium harbors the stem cells that are responsible for the proper epithelialization of the corneal surface. If a sufficient amount of limbal epithelium is destroyed, a state of limbal stem cell deficiency ensues. The result is the formation of persistent epithelial defects and/or the coverage, to a variable extent, of the corneal surface by conjunctival epithelium. Conjunctival epithelium is less transparent than corneal epithelium. It is also less adherent to the underlying corneal stroma; the resulting persistent epithelial defects are associated with chronic inflammation, neovascularization, scarring, ulceration, and melting (Figure 17-1). Limbal stem cell deficiency cannot be treated by penetrating keratoplasty since in conventional penetrating keratoplasty only central nonstem cells are transplanted.

The most common cause of limbal stem cell deficiency is chemical injury. However, there are a number of causes; these fall into three categories. The first is traumatic destruction of limbal stem cells as seen in chemical and thermal injury, multiple surgeries involving the limbal area, chronic contact lens-associated epitheliopathy (either as a result of the contact lenses themselves or the contact lens solutions), or chronic use of certain medications (such as 5-fluorouracil). The second category is the inflammatory destruction of limbal stem cells, as occurs in Stevens-Johnson syndrome and severe microbial keratitis. The third category is loss of limbal stem cells due to insufficient stromal support. This situation applies to aniridia and the keratitis associated with multiple endocrine neoplasia.

Conjunctivalization of the corneal surface is the most specific clinical sign of limbal stem cell deficiency. Conjunctival epithelium may be detected biomicroscopically by a dull or irregular reflex of the corneal surface. Staining with fluorescein produces a stippled pattern that is especially apparent after waiting a few minutes between application of fluorescein and viewing of the surface (ie, delayed staining). The more definitive way to diagnose limbal stem cell deficiency is by the identification of goblet cells on impression cytology (described in detail by Tseng). However, it is not practical (or necessary) to perform impression cytology on every patient with potential limbal stem cell deficiency, as long as one of the known causes of limbal stem cell deficiency is present and the patient exhibits the clinical signs of limbal stem cell deficiency.

Always Remember...

The most specific clinical sign of stem cell deficiency is conjunctivalization of the ocular surface detected by slit lamp examination, fluorescein staining characteristics, or impression cytology.

PEARL #72: OPTIMIZE THE OCULAR SURFACE

The success of limbal stem cell transplantation is strongly correlated with the extent to which the ocular surface environment has first been optimized (ie, the extent to which ocular surface abnormalities have been corrected). Specifically, sources of ongoing inflammation need to be eliminated or, if that is

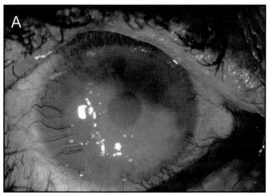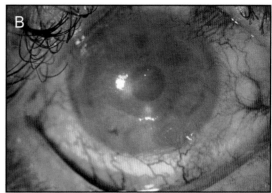

Figure 17-1 (Pearl 71). Limbal stem cell deficiency. This patient had sustained an acid splash to the right eye. The eye was copiously irrigated with saline at the time of injury and the patient treated with intensive topical corticosteroid medication, systemic ascorbate, and prophylactic antibiotic coverage. Limbal blanching indicative of limbal isch-emia was noted upon presentation. (A) Several months after the injury, the ocular surface demonstrates the effects of limbal stem cell deficiency with conjunctivalization of the surface and concomitant neovascularization, persistent epithelial defect formation, chronic inflammation, and stromal thinning. (B) The patient underwent limbal stem cell transplantation with donor tissue derived from his brother who represented a 100% HLA match. No systemic immunosuppression was utilized. Several months after transplantation, the cornea exhibits scarring, but there is no persistent epithelial defect, and the patient is significantly more comfortable. He is now ready for lamellar or penetrating keratoplasty.

not possible, addressed by immunomodulatory therapy (eg, dapsone and other agents in the case of ocular cicatricial pemphigoid). Infectious causes of inflammation need to be treated with anti-infectives and the use of potentially toxic topical medication minimized.

It is very important to pay attention to tear film, as well as eyelid and eyelash, abnormalities. Ocular surface dryness is addressed with preservative-free lubricating agents and punctal occlusion. Meibomian gland dysfunction is treated with warm compresses/lid hygiene and oral doxycycline (or similar medica-tion). Misdirected lashes are removed by electroepilation or some other means. Keratinization of the posterior lid margin is addressed with mucous membrane grafting. Excessive globe exposure is addressed with a permanent lateral tarsorrhaphy and eyelid malposition (such as entropion or ectropion) by plastic surgical interventions.

Eyes with extremely low Schirmer test values (less than 5 mm over 10 minutes) are eyes that are extremely difficult to rehabilitate regardless of the intervention instituted. In such a setting, salivary gland translocation microsurgery may hold some promise for those individuals whose salivary glands function normally. Tsubota and associates advocate the use of autologous serum eye drops in extreme dry eye situations such as those seen in Stevens-Johnson syndrome (Table 17-1, method of preparation).

Chemical injuries of the eye are a common cause of limbal stem cell deficiency states. Immediate treatment is geared toward controlling the pronounced inflammatory response typically accompanying this type of injury. These eyes are, therefore, treated with intensive topical corticosteroids, possibly an anticollagenolytic agent such as topical medroxyprogesterone, topical and systemic ascorbate, and pro-phylactic antibiotics. However, the point at which limbal stem cell transplantation should be pursued in cases associated with significant limbal stem cell damage is a source of controversy. Some authors advocate limbal stem cell transplantation at an early stage (ie, 2 to 3 weeks after injury). However, most authors feel that limbal stem cell transplantation should be delayed: the inflammation associated with the acute stage of a chemical injury as well as the presence of an ischemic limbal region makes survival of transplanted limbal stem cell tissue unlikely. Instead, such interventions as bandage contact lens place-ment, amniotic membrane transplantation (see Chapter 19), and tarsorrhaphy should be aggressively utilized to attempt reepithelialization. Limbal stem cell transplantation can then be performed at a later stage to rehabilitate a conjunctivalized and/or scarred corneal surface.

TABLE 17-1
HOW TO PREPARE AUTOLOGOUS SERUM EYE DROPS

1. Draw 50 cc of patient's blood in a red top test tube.
2. Centrifuge for 5 minutes at 1500 RPM. This will generally yield 25 cc of serum.
3. Aliquot 5 cc of the serum into five sterile tubes.
4. Dilute one of the five tubes with 20 cc of sterile balanced salt solution (producing a 20% serum solution).
5. Patient administers the drops four to six times per day using an eye dropper.
6. The solution is not preserved and needs to be stored in a refrigerator at 4° to 8°C. The remaining undiluted serum is frozen at -20°C until use.

Note:
1. Undiluted serum can also be used, but is very viscous.
2. Patients receiving serum eyedrops should also have punctal occlusion performed.

Adapted from Tsubota K, Goto E, Fujita H, et al. Treatment of dry eye by autologous serum application in Sjogren's syndrome. *Br J Ophthalmol.* 1999;83:390-395.

Always Remember...

Optimize the ocular surface prior to limbal stem cell transplantation: eliminate sources of inflammation/irritation, increase lubrication with punctal occlusion, and/or serum tears, and treat eyelid/eyelid position abnormalities.

In cases of chemical injury, do not place limbal stem cell grafts directly on a region of ischemic limbus. Delay limbal stem cell transplantation until revascularization of the limbus has occurred.

PEARL #73: LIMBAL STEM CELL AUTOGRAFTING: MAKE SURE THE CONTRALATERAL EYE IS NORMAL

Limbal stem cell autografting involves transplantation of limbal stem cell tissue from the unaffected eye of a patient to the affected eye and, therefore, is only performed in the setting of unilateral injury. Care should be taken to ascertain that the donor eye is truly normal, which sometimes can be difficult: an eye may appear normal but actually have a borderline limbal stem cell count. Patients may forget a previous injury or an injury may have actually been bilateral but asymmetric. Jenkins et al report a case of limbal stem cell deficiency occurring in a donor eye after limbal stem cell transplantation in a patient with contact lens related epitheliopathy. In this case, the donor eye probably was also affected but on initial inspection appeared normal. Others have reported similar cases.

Figures 17-2A and 17-2B illustrate preparation of the recipient eye. Abnormal tissue on the corneal surface is removed by blunt dissection utilizing tissue forceps and a surgical sponge (eg, a Merocel sponge [Medtronic Ophthalmics, Jacksonville, Fla]) and/or by sharp dissection utilizing a scarifier blade (eg, a Grieshaber or a Beaver 57 blade). Sharp dissection should be kept to a minimum since it carries the risk of corneal perforation and postoperative optical distortion from surface irregularity. Keeping the corneal surface dry often aids in identification of the correct tissue plane between superficial pannus and the underlying corneal stroma. A 360-degree conjunctival peritomy is performed and the conjunctiva recessed by a few millimeters. The conjunctival margins are secured with four interrupted 8-0 polyglactin (Vicryl [Ethicon, Somerville, NJ]) sutures, one in each quadrant. Some authors advocate performing a superficial sclerokeratectomy in order to create a bed for the donor tissue that minimizes a step-off at the edge of the tissue.

Donor tissue for limbal stem cell autografting is obtained as illustrated in Figure 17-2C. A maximum of 6 clock hours of limbal tissue is harvested either as two 3-clock hour segments or as three 2-clock hour segments. Each graft is harvested by first making a partial-thickness incision in the cornea approximately

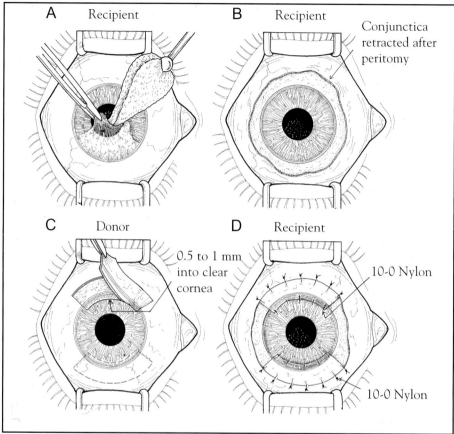

Figure 17-2 (Pearl 73). Limbal stem cell autografting. (A) Preparation of the recipient eye, part I. Abnormal tissue on the corneal surface is removed by blunt dissection. In this figure, use of tissue forceps and a surgical sponge (eg, a Merocel sponge) is illustrated. (B) Preparation of the recipient eye, part II. A 360-degree conjunctival peritomy and recession is performed. Some authors advocate performing a superficial sclerokeratectomy in order to create a bed for the donor tissue. (C) Harvesting of donor tissue. In this diagram, removal of two 3-clock hour segments of tissue is illustrated; three 2-clock hour segments may also be harvested. The cornea is incised 0.5 to 1 mm anterior to the limbus; see text for details. (D) Placement of donor tissue on the recipient bed. The donor tissue is secured with interrupted 10-0 nylon sutures.

0.5 to 1 mm anterior to the limbus for the appropriate width utilizing a blade. The second incision is made in the conjunctiva 2 mm posterior to the limbus with scissors. The conjunctiva is dissected up to its insertion at the limbus. The two incisions, conjunctival and corneal, are then joined by radial incisions at each end. The piece is lifted by the conjunctival edge and dissection carried anteriorly with the use of a crescent blade. Lamellar dissection of the cornea should be kept at a shallow level. The donor sites may be left open, although patients tend to be more comfortable if the sites are closed with Vicryl sutures.

The limbal stem cell grafts are sutured into place in the recipient bed (Figure 17-2D). The donor corneal edge of each graft is sutured to recipient cornea with interrupted 10-0 nylon sutures; likewise, the donor conjunctival edge is sutured to recipient sclera with interrupted 10-0 nylon sutures. The use of a fibrin sealant (eg, Tisseel VH [Baxter Healthcare Corp, Deerfield, Ill]) for securing the grafts has also been described. An overlay amniotic membrane patch may be placed to cover the cornea as well as the limbal stem cell grafts (see Chapter 19). A large-diameter, hydrophilic bandage contact lens (eg, a Kontur lens [Kontur, Richmond, Calif]) is placed at the end of the case for patient comfort and to

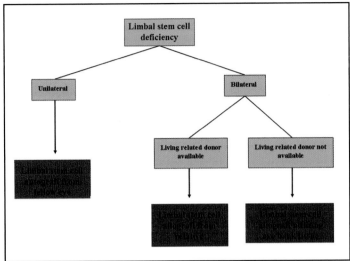

Figure 17-3 (Pearl 74). Algorithm for limbal stem cell transplantation. The evolution of epithelial transplantation for severe ocular surface disease and a proposed classification system. (Adapted from Holland EJ, Schwartz GS. The evolution of epithelial transplantation for severe ocular surface disease and a proposed classification system. *Cornea.* 1996;15:549-556.)

protect the transplanted tissue from the shearing effect of lid movements. A permanent lateral tarsorrhaphy is often performed in addition. Topical antibiotic and steroid medication is used until reepithelialization is complete and inflammation has subsided. Since limbal stem cell autografting involves only autologous tissue (ie, both donor and recipient tissue is from the same patient), systemic immunosuppression is not needed.

Always Remember…

Perform limbal stem cell autografting only in situations in which the donor eye is normal.

PEARL #74: LIMBAL STEM CELL ALLOGRAFTING: HUMAN LEUKOCYTE ANTIGEN TYPING AND POSTSURGICAL IMMUNOSUPPRESSION

If both eyes are affected, limbal stem cell allografting, in which limbal stem cell tissue is obtained either from an eye bank eye or from a living relative of the patient (living-related allograft), is necessary (Figure 17-3). Harvesting of limbal stem cell tissue from an eye bank eye is often referred to as keratolimbal allografting (KLAL) since, in this technique, the carrier tissue for the limbal stem cells is primarily corneal tissue. Harvesting of limbal stem cell tissue from a living-related donor is often called living-related conjunctival limbal allograft (lr-CLAL) since, in this technique, the carrier tissue for the limbal stem cells is primarily conjunctival tissue.

Recently, reports by Tsai et al, Schwab et al, and others describe the harvesting of small numbers of limbal stem cells from a patient, a patient's relative, or an eye bank eye. These cells are then expanded by culturing in the laboratory and then subsequently placed on the patient's eye utilizing amniotic membrane as a carrier tissue. This technique necessitates the removal of only a small amount of limbal tissue. Therefore, it would allow for the use, for example, of autologous tissue in settings in which there are only a small number of viable limbal stem cells remaining and in which currently allografting must be pursued. However, this technique is not yet widely available.

There is no consensus as to which type of allografting, living-related donor or eye bank donor, is superior. There are pros and cons to each. Tissue from a living donor is fresh tissue since it is transferred virtually immediately from donor to recipient eye while banked corneoscleral buttons are generally preserved for a few days in Optisol-GS (Bausch & Lomb, Rochester, NY) or similar medium. Use of eye bank tissue is also theoretically associated with a higher risk of rejection of the tissue (see following) since, in general, it is not practical to find eye bank tissue that provides a human leukocyte antigen

Figure 17-4 (Pearl 74). A typical immunosuppressive regimen.

Limbal Stem Cell Allografting:
Suggested Immunosuppression Regimen

Medications

- Prednisone   0.5 to 1 mg/kg/day
- Cyclosporine A (CsA)   3 mg/kg/day, in divided doses or a single daily dose
- Azathioprine   100 mg/day

Drug Monitoring

- Prednisone   Glucose at baseline and q 1 month while on substantial doses
- CsA   Creatinine at baseline and q 1 to 2 weeks
                                  CsA trough level maintained at 150 to 200 ng/mL
- Azathioprine   CBC, platelet count q 2 to 4 weeks

Clinical Follow-Up

- Prednisone   Tapered over 3 to 6 months (depending on level of inflammation) down to 10 to 15 mg/day. Continued for at least 12 months.
- CsA/Azathioprine   Continued for at least 12 months

Adapted from Holland EJ, Schwartz GS. Changing concepts in the management of severe ocular surface disease over twenty-five years. *Cornea* 2000;19:688.698.

(HLA) match to the patient. On the other hand, eye bank tissue is generally more readily available than living-related tissue. Furthermore, when using eye bank tissue, 360 degrees of limbal stem cell tissue can be harvested and placed on the recipient bed. This provides more limbal stem cells, and providing 360 degrees of limbal stem cell tissue theoretically creates a barrier effect to the inward migration of conjunctival tissue.

The corneal limbal area contains more antigen-presenting cells (eg, Langerhans cells) than does the central cornea. Therefore, the risk of rejection of the tissue is higher than for a typical penetrating keratoplasty. It is generally felt that HLA matching of tissue decreases the likelihood of rejection. However, unless tissue is found that is a perfect tissue-typing match to the recipient, systemic immunosuppression is probably still necessary in the setting of living-related allografting. It is always necessary in the setting of eye bank tissue allografting.

There is no consensus as to the optimal immunosuppression regimen or for how long immunosuppression should be continued. The topical agents typically used are corticosteroids and cyclosporine. The systemic agents typically utilized are prednisone and cyclosporine. A third systemic agent such as azathioprine, mycophenolate mofetil (eg, Cellcept [Roche, Nutley, NJ]), or tacrolimus (eg, Prograf [Fujisawa, Deerfield, Ill]) is sometimes used in addition. A typical immunosuppressive regimen is outlined in Figure 17-4. It is important to ensure there are no medical contraindications for use of these medications, and it is, therefore, critical for an ophthalmologist to work in concert with an internist when administering these medications.

Multiple studies have quoted success rates of 70% to 80% (as measured by development of a more normal corneal surface) for limbal stem cell allografting for a mean follow-up time of 1 to 2 years. However, this appears to fall to below 50% after 5 years. Holland and Schwartz divide limbal stem cell transplant failure into three categories. First is the type that develops immediately when transplantation is performed in an eye with persistent inflammation. In this type of a setting, there is direct damage to the transplanted tissue because of the inflammation. The second is the type that occurs in an eye that at baseline has minimal inflammation but that then develops an acute allograft rejection reaction as evidenced by intense vascular injection and edema at the graft-host junction and subsequent

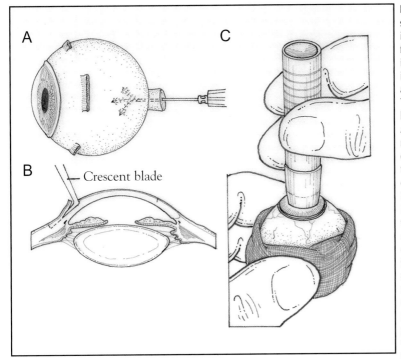

A

C

B — Crescent blade

Figure 17-5 (Pearl 74). Limbal stem cell allografting: harvesting donor limbal tissue from a fresh whole globe. (A) If the eye is overly soft, the eye can be injected with 1 to 2 mL of sterile air via the optic nerve stump. (B) The eye is wrapped in gauze and held by the optic nerve stump. A trephine with a diameter 3 mm smaller than the corneal diameter is used to create a partial-thickness trephination of the central cornea. (Adapted from Dua HS, Azuara-Blanco A. Allolimbal transplantation in patients with limbal stem cell deficiency. *Br J Ophthalmol* 1999;83:414-419.) (C) A crescent blade is used to perform a superficial lamellar dissection of the peripheral cornea to beyond the limbus and 1 mm into sclera. This results in removal of the endothelium and posterior corneoscleral tissue to yield a ring of limbal epithelium on a thin stromal carrier bed.

(Adapted from Foster CS, Mark DB. Corneoscleral lacerations and anterior segment reconstruction. In: Heilman K, Paton D, eds. *Atlas of Ophthalmic Surgery*. New York, NY: Theime; 1987;2:5.1-5.48.)

conjunctivalization of the ocular surface in the area of the rejection episode. Both the first and the second type warrant an increase in immunosuppressive therapy. The third type of failure is seen in a patient who initially has a successful limbal stem cell transplant who then goes on to develop a gradual, progressive conjunctivalization of the surface but without evidence of an increase in inflammation. This reaction represents either chronic, low-grade rejection or stem cell exhaustion.

The surgical technique for harvesting living-related donor tissue is identical to that of autografting. Ideally, simultaneous surgeries of the donor and recipient are scheduled in adjacent operating rooms. Once harvested, the limbal stem cell tissue is immediately placed into balanced salt solution and brought to the operating room suite of the recipient.

For allografting utilizing eye bank tissue, donor corneoscleral tissue can be obtained from either a fresh whole eye bank eye or a preserved corneoscleral "button." For a fresh whole eye, the eye is wrapped in gauze and held by the optic nerve stump (Figure 17-5). If the fresh eye is overly soft, the eye can be injected with 1 to 2 mL of sterile air via the optic nerve stump. A vacuum trephine with a diameter 3 mm smaller than the corneal diameter is then used to create a partial-thickness trephination of the central cornea. A crescent blade is used to perform a superficial lamellar dissection of the peripheral cornea to beyond the limbus and 1 mm into sclera. This results in removal of the endothelium and posterior stromal tissue to yield a ring of limbal epithelium on a thin stromal carrier bed. Additional tapering of the edges is performed to minimize development of a step-off when the tissue is placed on the recipient bed. The keratolimbal ring is then excised from the globe and sutured into place on the recipient eye as a circle or divided into half and sutured into place as two hemisegments. Interrupted 10-0 nylon sutures are used for both the corneal and the scleral edges.

If a corneoscleral button is used, the corneoscleral button is trimmed of excess scleral tissue and the central cornea removed with a trephine. A superficial lamellar dissection is then performed as described above and the harvested tissue is then sutured into place on the recipient eye (Figure 17-6). A corneoscleral rim can be challenging to work with. One approach is to place the rim on a petri dish

Figure 17-6 (Pearl 74). Limbal stem cell allografting using a corneoscleral button: placement of harvested corneoscleral hemisegments on recipient eye. The segments were obtained from an eye bank corneoscleral button as described in the text. In this case, three of four 180-degree segments obtained from two donor buttons were used. This provided the recipient eye with 1.5 times the transplanted limbal stem cells it would have received from a single donor eye. (Reprinted with permission from Holland EJ, Schwartz GS. Changing concepts in the management of severe ocular surface disease over twenty-five years. *Cornea.* 2000;19:688-698.)

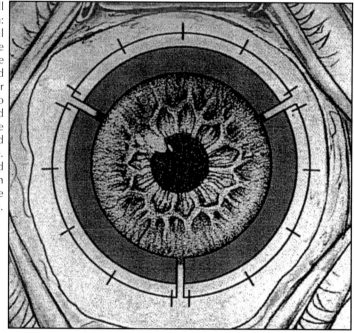

with the epithelial side facing down on a layer of viscoelastic. The rim is then thinned with the use of a blade and scissors: a blade can be used to first make a partial-thickness incision in the ring and this incision can then be used as an insertion point for the scissors. Mannis et al report a technique in which the corneoscleral button is supported on a standard silicone orbital sizing ball to provide a firm base for easier dissection of the tissue (Figure 17-7). The button is held in place on the ball with three 25-gauge needles; the hubs are removed with heavy scissors after the button has been secured to the ball. Meisler et al recently describe development of a suction device that does not rely on a freehanded technique of dissection of the keratolimbal ring. It is important during any dissection maneuver to protect the limbal epithelium as much as possible by gentle handling and liberal use of viscoelastic.

Always Remember...

Systemic immunosuppression is necessary in the case of limbal stem cell allografting.

Treat presumed limbal stem cell rejection with an increase in immunosuppressive therapy.

Protect limbal epithelium during surgical maneuvers with gentle handling and liberal use of viscoelastic.

PEARL #75: COMBINING LIMBAL STEM CELL TRANSPLANTATION AND CORNEAL GRAFTING: AT THE SAME TIME OR SPACED APART?

If scarring of the cornea is dense, visual rehabilitation usually requires performing a penetrating (or lamellar) keratoplasty in addition to limbal stem cell transplantation. The question is, should keratoplasty be performed at the same time as limbal stem cell transplantation or at a later time. In general, it is best to perform penetrating keratoplasty as a second procedure since the prognosis for penetrating keratoplasty improves as inflammation subsides and stromal neovascularization regresses. Furthermore, the corneal surface may improve after limbal stem cell transplantation to a sufficient degree to obviate the need for penetrating keratoplasty. Most authors recommend waiting a minimum of 3 months before proceeding with a penetrating keratoplasty.

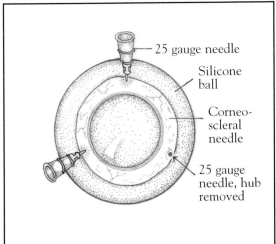

— 25 gauge needle

Silicone
ball

Corneo-
scleral
needle

25 gauge
needle, hub
removed

Figure 17-7 (Pearl 74). Limbal stem cell allografting: harvesting of donor limbal tissue from a corneoscleral button. To facilitate handling of a corneoscleral button, the button is supported on a standard silicone-sizing ball. The button is held in place on the ball with three 25-gauge needles; the hubs are removed with heavy scissors after the button has been secured to the ball. (Adapted from Mannis MJ, McCarthy M, Izquierdo L. Technique for harvesting keratolimbal allografts from corneoscleral buttons. *Am J Ophthalmol.* 1999;128:237-238.)

One advantage associated with performing limbal stem cell transplantation and penetrating keratoplasty simultaneously is that in the case of limbal stem cell allografting, both the limbal tissue and corneal tissue are generally from the same donor. Therefore, there is foreign antigenic presentation to the recipient from only one donor source. It is not known whether this makes a difference in regard to rejection risk.

One approach to performing a simultaneous limbal stem cell transplant and penetrating keratoplasty is described by Tseng et al. The recipient bed is prepared in the manner described in Pearl #74. The central cornea is then removed from the recipient with a 7.75-mm trephine. An 8.0-mm donor corneal button is then sutured to the recipient bed with eight cardinal interrupted 10-0 nylon sutures. The donor corneolimbal ring is then thinned as described in Pearl #75 and transferred to the recipient eye. The scleral edge is secured to the recipient sclera with interrupted 10-0 nylon sutures. The corneal edge is secured to the donor corneal button with eight interrupted 10-0 nylon sutures, which are passed to include portions of donor corneal button, recipient peripheral cornea, and donor corneolimbal ring. The first set of eight sutures placed is then removed. The donor cornea is then secured with an additional 16-bite running 10-0 nylon suture. An altogether alternate approach to a simultaneous limbal stem cell/corneal transplant is described by Reinhard et al. This approach involves performing an eccentric trephination of a corneoscleral button such that 30% to 40% of the circumference of the button contains limbal tissue.

Always Remember…

In general, perform limbal stem cell transplantation and lamellar/penetrating keratoplasty as staged procedures.

BIBLIOGRAPHY

Dogru M, Tsubota K. Current concepts in ocular surface reconstruction. *Semin Ophthalmol.* 2005;20:75-93.

Dua HS, Azuara-Blanco A. Allo-limbal transplantation in patients with limbal stem cell deficiency. *Br J Ophthalmol.* 1999;83:414-419.

Holland EJ, Schwatrz GS. Changing concepts in the management of severe ocular surface disease over twenty-five years. *Cornea.* 2000;19:688-698.

Jenkins C, Tuft S, Liu C, et al. Limbal transplantation in the management of chronic contact lens-associated epitheliopathy. *Eye.* 1993;7:629-633.

Kenyon KR, Tseng SCG. Limbal autograft transplantation for ocular surface disorders. *Ophthalmology.* 1989;96:709-723.

Meisler DM, Perez VL, Proudfit J. A device to facilitate limbal stem cell procurement from eye bank donor tissue for keratolimbal allograft procedures. *Am J Ophthalmol.* 2005;139:212-214.

Rao SK, Rajagopal R, Sitalakshmi G, et al. Limbal allografting from related live donors for corneal surface reconstruction. *Ophthalmology.* 1999;106:822-828.

Reinhard T, Spelsberg H, Henke L. Long-term results of allogeneic penetrating limbo-keratoplasty in total limbal stem cell deficiency. *Ophthalmology.* 2004;111:775-782.

Samson CM, Nduaguba C, Baltatzis S, Foster CS. Limbal stem cell transplantation in chronic inflammatory disease. *Ophthalmology.* 2002;109:862-868.

Schwab IR, Reyes M, Isseroff RR. Successful transplantation of bioengineered tissue replacements in patients with ocular surface disease. *Cornea.* 2000;19:421-426.

Solomon A, Ellies P, Anderson DF, et al. Long-term outcome of keratolimbal allograft for total limbal stem cell deficiency. *Ophthalmology.* 2002;109:1159-1166.

Tan DTH, Ficker LA, Buckley RJ. Limbal transplantation. *Ophthalmology.* 1996;103:29-36.

Tsai R J-F, Tseng SCG. Effect of stromal inflammation on the outcome of limbal transplantation for corneal surface reconstruction. *Cornea.* 1995;14:439-449.

Tsai R J-F, Li L-M, Chen J-K. Reconstruction of damaged corneas by transplantation of autologous limbal epithelial cells. *N Engl J Med.* 2000;343:86-93.

Tseng SCG. Staging of conjunctival metaplasia by impression cytology. *Ophthalmology.* 1985;6:728-733.

Tseng SCG, Prabhasawat P, Barton K, et al. Amniotic membrane transplantation with or without limbal allografts for corneal surface reconstruction in patients with limbal stem cell deficiency. *Arch Ophthalmol.* 1998;116:431-441.

Tsubota K, Satake Y, Kaido M, et al. Treatment of severe ocular surface disorders with corneal epithelial stem cell transplantation. *N Engl J Med.* 1999;340:1697-1703.

CHAPTER 18

Two
Pearls for Successful Pterygium Excision

Tushar Agarwal, MD; Namrata Sharma, MD; and Rasik B. Vajpayee, MS, FRCSEd

Treatment of a symptomatic pterygium ranges from a single definitive procedure to a combination of strategies to combat recurring aggressive disease. These include beta-irradiation, MMC application, and conjunctival and amniotic membrane grafting. In this chapter, we describe surgical techniques that may improve the cosmetic success of the excision as well as decrease the rate of recurrence.

Pearl #76: Mitomycin C: Pros and Cons

Topical application of MMC is one of the most commonly used adjunctive therapies employed to check the recurrence of a pterygium. Others include chemotherapy (thiotepa) and radiation therapy. MMC use with pterygium surgery was popularized in the United States by Singh et al. The drug may be applied locally on the sclera for 1 to 3 minutes at the site of excised pterygium or used as topical drops postoperatively for a short cycle treatment. The optimal dosage of mitomycin to be used to prevent recurrence is not clear, but the risk of complications is believed to be reduced if postoperative application is avoided.

The standard technique employs the use of a cellulose sponge or a filter paper that has been cut to the size of the sclera bared by the pterygium excision and has been soaked in 0.02% MMC. The sponge is placed on the bare sclera for 1 to 3 minutes after the pterygium has been excised. This is followed by copious irrigation to remove any remnants of the toxic drug. MMC is capable of causing toxicity, and the common complication is that of localized scleral melting. Figure 18-1 shows corneoscleral melting after MMC use as topical drops following pterygium excision. If scleral melting occurs, it is advisable to send scleral scrapings for cultures to rule out a microbial super infection. If the melting is severe, a scleral patch graft may be required to strengthen the thinned scleral tissue. Other complications include severe glaucoma, corneal edema and perforation, correctopia, cataract formation, photophobia, and pain.

Always Remember...

Scleral melting is not always related to mitomycin C application. It is advisable to obtain scleral scrapings for cultures to rule out microbial super infection.

Pearl #77: Cosmetic Autografts with Fibrin Tissue Glue

Conjunctival autografting has emerged as an effective surgical modality, especially in cases of recurrent pterygia. The superior cosmetic result as compared to bare sclera techniques has made this procedure widely popular. The improved cosmetic result is related to the removal of the inflamed conjunctival tissue without leaving an avascular white scleral patch, usually seen after the use of either mitomycin or beta radiation. Preliminary data on amniotic membrane gluing instead of autografts shows further reduction in surgical time but possibly a higher rate of recurrence.

A thorough, meticulous dissection and removal of the subconjunctival tissue beneath the pterygium is the first step toward increasing the success rate of pterygium surgery. Excision of 1 to 2 mm of subconjunctival tissue peripheral to the areas surrounding the excised pterygium may provide better

Figure 18-1 (Pearl 76). Corneoscleral melting after mitomycin C use as topical drops following pterygium excision.

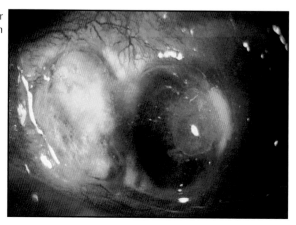

Figure 18-2 (Pearl 77). Conjunctival graft harvesting. Balanced salt solution or lidocaine is injected as soon as the tip of the needle perforates the conjunctiva to separate it from the underlying tissue plane.

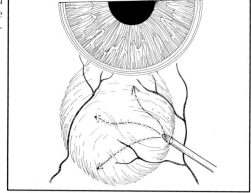

protection against recurrence. In cases of a recurrent and/or aggressive pterygium, the subconjunctival tissue is very thick and fibrosed and may be merged with the insertion of the horizontal rectus muscle. In such cases, the muscle should be identified and isolated with a Vicryl suture at its insertion to avoid inadvertent injury.

The conjunctival graft is usually harvested from the upper temporal area of the same eye that is undergoing pterygium surgery. Corneal traction sutures can be used to tort the globe inferiorly, providing good exposure. Alternatively, the graft may be harvested from the other eye. The bare area is measured to harvest a corresponding-sized autograft. Gentian violet can be used to mark the area to be excised and help preserve the upside-down orientation. Balanced salt solution or 2% lidocaine with epinephrine is then injected in the subconjunctival space starting outside the marked area. It is important to separate the conjunctiva from the underlying subconjunctival tissue and Tenon's capsule because this will affect the cosmetic appearance and the postoperative tissue shrinkage. This is made easier with injection of the anesthetic as soon as the tip of the needle penetrates the conjunctiva (Figure 18-2). Gentle tissue handling is crucial to avoid shredding of the graft tissue. We suggest a no-touch technique through a 3-mm opening created at the edge of the ballooned conjunctiva through which scissors are introduced to sever the subconjunctival adhesions without the need to hold the edge of the tissue. Care should also be taken to avoid any perforation of the conjunctival tissue. Tenon's capsule adheres tightly to the overlying conjunctival tissue at the limbus and can be separated by gentle dissection while reflecting the conjunctival flap over the cornea. The graft is then excised and transferred toward the bare scleral area. Copious irrigation of the conjunctival graft throughout the dissection procedure will ensure against tissue shrinkage. The correct vertical orientation should be preserved. It is especially important to firmly grasp the conjunctival graft when releasing the traction sutures, allowing the globe to rotate upward without disturbing the tissue orientation. If the latter is disrupted, the epithelial surface may be identified because it has a tendency to roll at the edges toward the posterior surface.

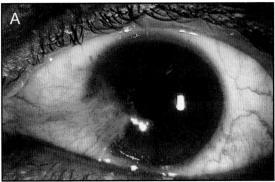 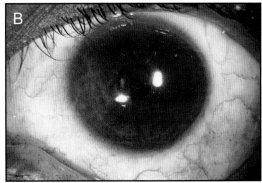

Figure 18-3 (Pearl 77). (A) The preoperative appearance of a case of advanced pterygium. (B) The postoperative appearance of the same eye after pterygium excision and conjunctival autograft.

The autograft is then sutured to the edges of the cut conjunctiva using either a 10-0 nylon or an 8-0 Vicryl suture. To prevent the sliding of the graft, it is preferable to anchor it to the scleral bed in a few locations. Alternatively, Tisseel Duo Quick (Baxter, Vienna, Austria), which is a tissue adhesive that mimics the natural fibrin formation, can also be used to attach the graft to the bare sclera. Use of this glue instead of sutures is reported to cause significantly less postoperative pain and shortens surgery time. Figure 18-3A shows the preoperative appearance of a case of advanced pterygium. Figure 18-3B shows the postoperative appearance of the same eye after pterygium excision and conjunctival autograft. Figure 18-4 also shows pre- and postoperative pictures of pterygium excision with conjunctival autograft.

In the early postoperative period, we advocate liberal use of topical antibiotic-steroid ointment combination (eg, TobraDex [Alcon Surgical, Fort Worth, Tex]). Figure 18-5 shows postoperative results with use of Tisseel glue.

Always Remember…

Copious, continuous irrigation of the conjunctival graft throughout the dissection procedure will ensure against tissue shrinkage.

When using premixed Tisseel fibrin glue, time is of the essence. Injecting the mixture under the positioned graft may result in excess glue amount, which may require immediate attention.

Application of the fibrin glue may be easier if the fibrinogen and the thrombin components are applied separately on the graft and sclera respectively.

BIBLIOGRAPHY

Basti S, Rao SK. Current status of limbal conjunctival autograft. *Curr Opin Ophthalmol.* 2000;11(4):224-232.

Coroneo MT, Di Girolamo N, Wakefield D. The pathogenesis of pterygia. *Curr Opin Ophthalmol.* 1999;10(4):282-288.

Hardten DR, Samuelson TW. Ocular toxicity of mitomycin-C. *Int Ophthalmol Clin.* 1999;39(2):79-90.

Hoffman RS, Power WJ. Current options in pterygium management. *Int Ophthalmol Clin.* 1999;39(1):15-26.

Kenyon KR, Wagoner MD, Hettinger ME. Conjunctival autograft transplantation for advanced and recurrent pterygium. *Ophthalmology.* 1985;92(11):1461-1470.

Koranyi G, Seregard S, Kopp ED. Cut and paste: a no suture, small incision approach to pterygium surgery. *Br J Ophthalmol.* 2004;88(7):911-914.

Singh G, Wilson MR, Foster CS. Mitomycin eye drops as treatment for pterygium. *Ophthalmology.* 1988;95(6):813-821.

Singh G, Wilson MR, Foster CS. Long-term follow-up study of mitomycin eye drops as adjunctive treatment of pterygia and its comparison with conjunctival autograft transplantation. *Cornea.* 1990;9(4):331-334.

Starck T, Kenyon KR, Serrano F. Conjunctival autograft for primary and recurrent pterygia: surgical technique and problem management. *Cornea.* 1991;10(3):196-202.

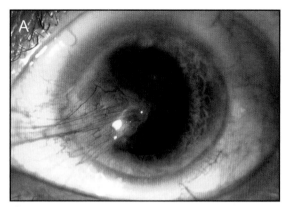

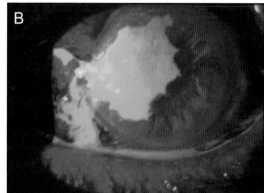

Figure 18-4 (Pearl 77). (A, B, C) Pre- and postoperative pictures of pterygium excision with conjunctival autograft. (Courtesy of Samir A. Melki, MD, PhD.)

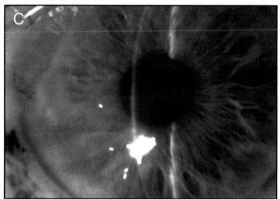

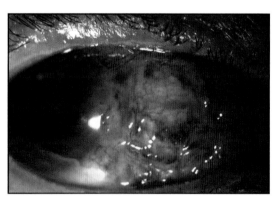

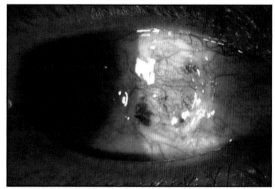

Figure 18-5 (Pearl 77). Postoperative results with use of fibrin glue. (Courtesy of Samir A. Melki, MD, PhD.)

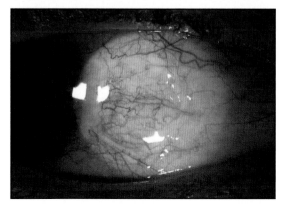

CHAPTER 19

THREE
PEARLS IN AMNIOTIC MEMBRANE
TRANSPLANTATION

Kimberly C. Sippel, MD and C. Stephen Foster, MD, FACS

PEARL #78: AMNIOTIC MEMBRANE TRANSPLANTATION: WHEN WOULD ONE CONSIDER USING IT?

Human placental amnion consists of a single epithelial layer, a basement membrane, and an avascular stroma (Figure 19-1). Amniotic membrane has a number of properties that are useful in the setting of ocular surface reconstruction: the membrane provides a stable substrate for epithelialization in situations, for example, in which there is damage to the corneal epithelial basement membrane and/or underlying stroma; it seems capable of discouraging fibrovascular ingrowth, inflammatory cell infiltration, and abnormal neovascularization; and the epithelium elaborates growth factors beneficial to the epithelialization process. Of note, it does not constitute a permanent replacement for epithelial tissue (whether corneal or conjunctival) since it is absorbed after several weeks. Furthermore, it is not capable of providing significant tectonic support.

Numerous clinical indications for the use of amniotic membrane transplantation have been described. One application is to facilitate epithelialization of persistent epithelial defects with or without sterile ulceration that have failed more conservative interventions such as elimination of toxic topical medications, lubrication, punctal occlusion, bandage contact lens placement, or tarsorrhaphy. A second setting in which amniotic membrane transplantation has been used is in the acute stages of severe chemical or thermal injury, Stevens-Johnson syndrome, and toxic epidermal necrolysis in order to promote reepithelialization and minimize symblepharon formation.

Amniotic membrane can also be used as a temporary replacement for conjunctival tissue. For example, it can be used to cover an area of bare sclera after the excision of a large ocular surface neoplasm as long as there is an adjacent area of normal conjunctiva to serve as a source of conjunctival epithelial cells for permanent coverage. Amniotic membrane transplantation can also take the place of conjunctival autografting in the setting of pterygium surgery. This is especially useful if there is minimal normal conjunctival tissue available or if there is a possible need for a future glaucoma filtering procedure.

Amniotic membrane transplantation has also been used to aid ocular surface reconstruction in the setting of limbal stem cell deficiency states such as those resulting from chemical injury or ocular cicatrizing conditions (eg, ocular cicatricial pemphigoid or Stevens-Johnson syndrome). In cases of partial limbal stem cell deficiency, amniotic membrane alone may be used: it has been postulated that amniotic membrane may allow for maximization of the function of the remaining limbal stem cells. However, if a state of total limbal stem cell deficiency exists, amniotic membrane transplantation alone will not be successful. In this setting, amniotic membrane transplantation needs to be combined with limbal stem cell transplantation (see Chapter 17).

Most recently, amniotic membrane has been used as a carrier tissue to transfer cultivated limbal epithelial cells (which are presumed to be limbal stem cells) onto the ocular surface to treat conditions involving limbal stem cell deficiency.

Figure 19-1 (Pearl 78). The three layers of amniotic membrane. Amniotic membrane is oriented on nitrocellulose paper in such a way that the epithelium/basement membrane side faces up. The epithelium/basement membrane side tends to be less sticky than the stromal side, a feature that aids in correctly orienting the tissue.

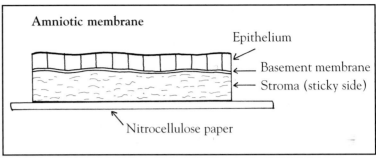

Always Remember...

In ocular surface reconstruction, it is critical to first optimize the ocular surface with such interventions as lubrication and punctal occlusion, use of preservative-free medications, treatment of meibomian gland dysfunction, lateral tarsorrhaphy or other lid tightening procedures, as well as mucous membrane grafting, if necessary.

Amniotic membrane transplantation alone cannot correct a state of total limbal stem cell deficiency.

PEARL #79: AMNIOTIC MEMBRANE TRANSPLANTATION: WHERE DOES ONE OBTAIN AMNIOTIC MEMBRANE?

One common method of preparation of amniotic membrane is described by Lee and Tseng. Human placenta is obtained shortly after elective cesarean delivery. The mother is confirmed to be negative for human immunodeficiency virus, human T-lymphocyte virus, hepatitis virus types B and C, and syphilis both at the time of procurement and then 6 months later. The amniotic membrane is then separated from the rest of the chorion by blunt dissection and then flattened onto nitrocellulose paper with the epithelium/basement membrane side up (away from the filter paper). The filter paper is then cryopreserved by storage at –80°C in Dulbecco modified Eagle medium and glycerol (at a ratio of 1:1 [v/v]) containing penicillin, streptomycin, neomycin, and amphotericin B.

Amniotic membrane is also commercially available in the United States. It can be ordered in a cryopreserved state from Bio-Tissue, Inc (Miami, Fla) or in a dehydrated state from Innovative Ophthalmic Products, Inc (Costa Mesa, Calif). To date, there have been no comparative clinical trials to determine if either preparation (cryopreserved or dehydrated) offers superior efficacy.

Cryopreserved amniotic membrane can be stored at –80°C for at least 1 year. It is shipped overnight on dry ice and can then be stored at –20°C (a regular freezer) for up to 3 months or in a refrigerator at 4°C for 1 week. It should be brought to room temperature only 5 to 10 minutes before use. If the thawed membrane is not used, it may be placed back in a freezer for future use as long as the bottle was not opened.

Dehydrated amniotic membrane lasts a couple of years at room temperature. When it is ready to be used, it can first be trimmed to the size needed in its dry state. It is then applied to the surgical site and rehydrated by placing drops of saline on the membrane and then waiting 5 to 10 minutes. Care must be taken to fully rehydrate the tissue. The indication that the tissue has been properly rehydrated is that the grid pattern of the membrane (visible under magnification) disappears.

The amniotic epithelium elaborates a host of growth factors that are probably beneficial for the process of epithelialization. Although one report suggests the amniotic epithelium may survive up to 70 days after cryopreservation, it is unclear how well (and for how long) the amniotic epithelium (and associated growth factors) survives cryopreservation. However, use of fresh amniotic membrane is generally impractical and does not allow for the adequate safeguarding against the transmission of blood-borne illnesses. Most studies involving amniotic membrane transplantation utilized cryopreserved membrane and have confirmed that amniotic membrane confers beneficial effects even after cryopreservation.

Recently, Bio-Tissue has begun to offer a sutureless amniotic membrane option called Prokera. Prokera consists of a sheet of amniotic membrane placed within an ophthalmic conformer ring. This device can then be applied to the eye in an office setting, without the need for sutures, and functions effectively as an amniotic membrane overlay patch (see below).

Always Remember…

Be sure to sufficiently rehydrate dehydrated amniotic membrane.

PEARL #80: INLAY OR OVERLAY?

Corneal Defects

There are two ways in which amniotic membrane may be applied to the ocular surface: using an inlay technique or using an overlay technique. In the inlay method, also known as the graft method, amniotic membrane is sized to fit the size of the defect. In this setting, it is presumed the amniotic membrane serves as a substrate over which the new corneal epithelium grows. In general, the inlay method is used if the corneal basement membrane is damaged and/or there is loss of corneal stromal substrate. In the overlay, or patch, technique amniotic membrane is placed over the entire cornea, limbus, and perilimbal area. When applied in this manner, the amniotic membrane functions essentially as a biological contact lens. If necessary, both techniques can be utilized in the same eye (ie, first, an inlay graft is placed; a second amniotic membrane sheet is then placed in an overlay fashion).

Abnormal tissue is first debrided from the corneal surface by blunt dissection utilizing, for example, tissue forceps and a surgical sponge (eg, a Merocel sponge [Medtronic Ophthalmics, Jacksonville, Fla]). Keeping the corneal surface dry often aids in identification of the correct tissue plane between superficial pannus and the underlying corneal stroma. If cryopreserved membrane is used, the amniotic membrane is thawed, peeled off the nitrocellulose filter paper, placed onto the recipient area, and then trimmed to size with scissors. It may be, but does not have to be, rinsed with saline. If dehydrated amniotic membrane is used, the membrane is applied as described under Pearl #80.

In the inlay technique, it is important to orient the amniotic membrane with the stromal side facing down; orientation is less critical in the overlay method. There are several ways to know which side is the stromal side. First, cryopreserved membrane is oriented on the nitrocellulose paper with the stromal side down on the filter paper. Dehydrated amniotic membrane has a grid texture before rehydration: the stromal side is the convex, or elevated, side of the grid. Second, the stromal side is stickier than the basement membrane side. Stickiness can be assessed with the use of a surgical sponge such as a Merocel sponge. Furthermore, a fine strand of vitreous-like substance can typically be drawn up from the stromal side but not from the epithelial side.

In the inlay method (Figure 19-2), the amniotic membrane is cut to be somewhat larger than the size of the defect. In the case of a corneal lesion such as a persistent epithelial defect, the membrane is secured to the edge of the defect with interrupted 9-0 or 10-0 polyglactin (Vicryl [Ethicon, Somerville, NJ]) or 10-0 nylon sutures. These may be placed radially, as seen in Figure 19-2, or parallel to the cut edge of the amniotic membrane. Alternatively, one anchoring suture is placed, followed by a running suture. It is best not to trim the amniotic membrane to the exact size of the defect at the beginning but to trim as one goes along since the membrane may shrink to some extent. An additional second sheet of amniotic membrane may be placed in an overlay fashion.

In the case of deep stromal ulceration, more than one layer of amniotic membrane can be used to fill the ulcer crater. This layering may be achieved either by folding a sheet of amniotic membrane multiple times like a blanket or by folding it accordion style. Orientation of the layers (whether the stromal side is up or down) is not critical for these layers. These layers are not sutured. Finally, an additional sheet of amniotic membrane is placed in an overlay fashion and sutured in place.

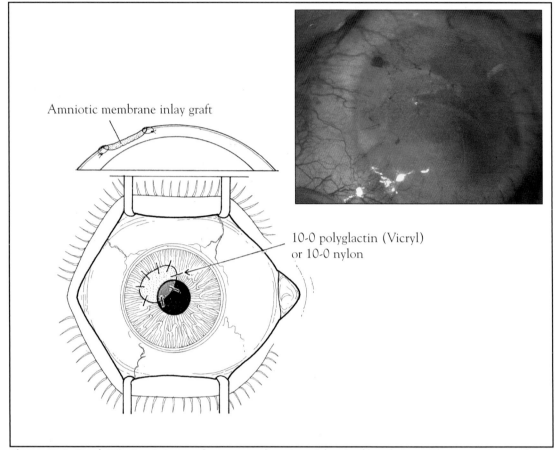

Figure 19-2 (Pearl 80). Amniotic membrane transplantation, inlay (graft) technique. The amniotic membrane is sized to the defect and then secured to the cornea with interrupted 9-0 or 10-0 polyglactin (Vicryl) or 10-0 nylon sutures. The sutures may be radial, as illustrated in the figure, or parallel to the cut edge of the membrane. Alternatively, a running suture may be utilized. The inset photograph depicts an amniotic membrane inlay graft in a patient who developed a neurotrophic ulcer after undergoing a penetrating keratoplasty. The ulcer did not respond to lubrication or bandage contact lens placement. In this case, the amniotic membrane graft was secured with radial 10-0 Vicryl suture.

In the overlay method (Figure 19-3), the amniotic membrane is cut 14 to 16 mm diameter in size and used to cover the entire corneal, limbal, and perilimbal area. The membrane is secured to the surrounding conjunctiva with interrupted 8-0 Vicryl sutures utilizing bites that include the episclera. If necessary, an additional purse-string or series of interrupted 10-0 nylon sutures parallel to the limbus may be placed in the peripheral cornea to further secure the membrane.

If amniotic membrane transplantation is combined with limbal stem cell transplantation, the limbal stem cell grafts are first sutured into place, and amniotic membrane is then placed utilizing the overlay technique. However, if the corneal surface is markedly irregular and the corneal basement membrane significantly damaged, an inlay amniotic membrane graft may be placed first (stromal side down) and then the limbal stem cell grafts placed on top. An additional overlay amniotic membrane may then be placed.

Afterwards, a large-diameter, hydrophilic bandage contact lens is applied (eg, Kontur lens). Topical antibiotic and steroid medication is used until reepithelialization is complete and inflammation has subsided. Since amniotic membrane epithelium typically does not survive the preservation process, amniotic membrane is not antigenic, and therefore, immunosuppression is not necessary. The amniotic membrane dissolves under the bandage contact lens over a period of a few weeks. Residual nylon suture

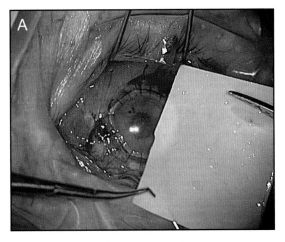

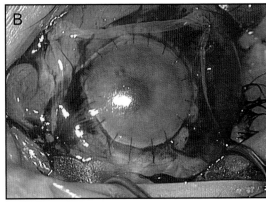

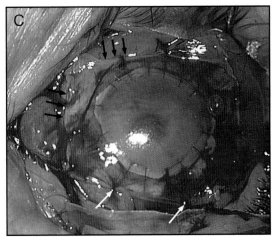

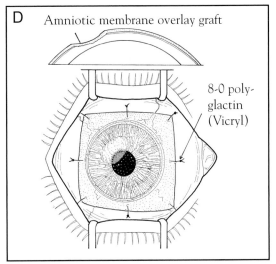

Figure 19-3 (Pearl 80). Amniotic membrane transplantation, overlay (patch) technique. The patient underwent a lamellar keratoplasty for a large pterygium. As a result of the large size of the pterygium, the patient was felt to have a significant, although not total, limbal stem cell deficiency in the involved eye. Overlay amniotic membrane transplantation was performed to maximize function of the remaining limbal stem cells. (A) The amniotic membrane is cut to approximately 14 to 16 mm in diameter and then peeled off the nitrocellulose paper. (B) The amniotic membrane sheet is placed on the eye. The 10-0 nylon sutures visible here are those securing the lamellar graft and are not directly related to the amniotic membrane transplant. (C) The amniotic membrane sheet is secured to the conjunctiva/episclera with interrupted 8-0 Vicryl sutures. The black arrows delineate the edge of the amniotic membrane sheet. The white arrows highlight the positions of two representative 8-0 Vicryl sutures. (D) Schematic representation of an overlay amniotic membrane transplant.

(if used) may be removed after healing has taken place. When used as an inlay graft on the cornea, the amniotic membrane may become incorporated to some extent into the substance of the cornea, leading potentially to a slight loss of corneal transparency, which may persist for some time.

A dry ocular surface and/or an excessively exposed globe will hasten dissolution of amniotic membrane. Therefore, addressing dryness and exposure issues will allow the membrane to remain on the eye for a longer period. Therefore, this often necessitates concomitant performance of punctal occlusion and/or a lateral tarsorhaphy. Repeat applications of amniotic membrane may also be necessary.

Conjunctival Defects

For conjunctival defects created after pterygium excision or after removal of an ocular surface neoplasm, the inlay method of amniotic membrane transplantation is generally utilized. The amniotic

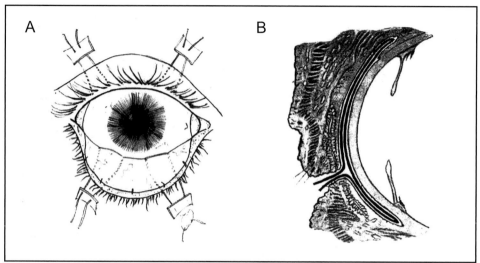

Figure 19-4 (Pearl 80). Use of amniotic membrane in the setting of acute chemical/thermal injury or Stevens-Johnson syndrome/toxic epidermal necrolysis. To minimize the risk of symblepharon formation, a large sheet of amniotic membrane is used to cover the entire ocular surface and then sutured close to the edges of both upper and lower eyelids. (A) To protect the depth of the fornices, the amniotic membrane is secured with two double-armed horizontal mattress sutures of 6-0 silk, brought temporally and nasally through full-thickness lid and tied over the skin with bolsters. (B) Cross-sectional view demonstrating how amniotic membrane covers the entire ocular surface from the upper lid margin to the lower lid margin. (Reprinted with permission from Elsevier; Meller D, Pires RTF, Mack RJS, et al. Amniotic membrane transplantation for acute chemical or thermal burns. *Ophthalmology.* 2000;107(5):980-990.

membrane is sized to fit the conjunctival defect and then sutured into place with interrupted 8-0 Vicryl sutures.

In situations of acute ocular chemical or thermal injury in which a large area of conjunctival tissue is typically affected and the demarcation of intact and damaged conjunctiva often not well-defined, the overlay technique is generally utilized. To decrease the risk of symblepharon formation, a large sheet of amniotic membrane is sutured close to the edges of both upper and lower eyelids with interrupted 9-0 or 10-0 Vicryl or 10-0 nylon sutures, thus covering the entire ocular surface. Placement of the lid sutures is facilitated by eversion of the lid with a chalazion clamp. To protect the depth of the fornices, the amniotic membrane is secured with two double-armed horizontal mattress sutures of 6-0 silk brought temporally and nasally through full-thickness lid and tied over the skin with bolsters (Figure 19-4). As mentioned above, in the case of severe chemical burns associated with total limbal stem cell deficiency, amniotic membrane transplantation alone may reduce conjunctival scarring and enhance corneal reepithelialization but does not prevent the sequelae of limbal stem cell deficiency.

Always Remember...

A 1:1000 dilution of epinephrine can be used at the start of a surgical procedure involving extensive corneal pannus dissection to induce vasoconstriction and decrease bleeding.

Amniotic membrane may be applied utilizing an inlay, or graft, technique or an overlay, or patch, technique.

A dry ocular surface and/or exposure will cause amniotic membrane to dissolve excessively quickly.

BIBLIOGRAPHY

Dua, HS, Gomes JAP, King AJ, Maharajan VS. The amniotic membrane in ophthalmology. *Surv Ophthalmol.* 2004;49:51-77.

Fernandes M, Sridhar MS, Sangwan VS, Rao GN. Amniotic membrane transplantation for ocular surface reconstruction. *Cornea.* 2005;24:643-653.

Hanada K, Shimazaki J, Shimmura S, Tsubota K. Multilayered amniotic membrane transplantation for severe ulceration of the cornea and sclera. *Am J Ophthalmol.* 2001;131:324-331.

Honaver SG, Bansal AK, Sangwan VS, Rao GN. Amniotic membrane for ocular surface reconstruction in Stevens-Johnson syndrome. *Ophthalmology.* 2000;107975-979.

John T, Foulks GN, John ME, Cheng K, Hu D. Amniotic membrane in the surgical management of acute toxic epidermal necrolysis. *Ophthalmology.* 2002;109:351-360.

Kruse FE, Rohrschneider K, Volcker HE. Multilayer amniotic membrane transplantation for reconstruction of deep corneal ulcers. *Ophthalmology.* 1999;106:1504-1511.

Lee SH, Tseng SCG. Amniotic membrane transplantation for persistent epithelial defects with ulceration. *Am J Ophthalmol.* 1997;123:303-312.

Letko E, Stechschulte SU, Kenyon KR, et al. Amniotic membrane inlay and overlay grafting for corneal epithelial defects and stromal ulcers. *Arch Ophthalmol.* 2001;119:659-63.

Meller D, Pires RTF, Mack RJS, et al. Amniotic membrane transplantation for acute chemical or thermal burns. *Ophthalmology.* 2000;107:980-990.

Prabhasawat P, Barton K, Burkett G, Tseng SCG. Comparison of conjunctival autografts, amniotic membrane grafts, and primary closure for pterygium excision. *Ophthalmology.* 1997;104:974-985.

Shimazaki J, Yang HY, Tsubota K. Amniotic membrane transplantation for ocular surface reconstruction in patients with chemical and thermal burns. *Ophthalmology.* 1997;104:2068-76.

Shimazaki J, Shinozaki N, Tsubota K. Transplantation of amniotic membrane and limbal autograft for patients with recurrent pterygium associated with symblepharon. *Br J Ophthalmol.* 1998;82:235-240.

Tseng SC, Prabhasawat P, Lee SH. Amniotic membrane transplantation with or without limbal allografts for corneal surface reconstruction in patients with limbal stem cell deficiency. *Am J Ophthalmol.* 1997;124:765-774.

CHAPTER 20

THREE
PEARLS FOR SUTURING CORNEAL INCISIONS AND LACERATIONS

Roberto Pineda II, MD

This chapter will review important principles in suturing corneal incisions and lacerations. In addition to restoration of corneal sphericity, the goal of corneal laceration repair should always include release of uveal and vitreous incarceration, prevention and management of infections, and preparation for secondary repair. Minimizing induced astigmatism is especially important for corneal lacerations greater than 4 mm in length or more than one-third the corneal diameter because these lacerations have been shown to result in greater amounts of astigmatism and poorer visual outcomes. The recommendations presented here will help manage traumatic refractive astigmatism at the time of the surgical repair and aid in reconstitution of a spherical cornea. Applying these pearls will result in the best potential outcome in both the short and long term.

PEARL # 81: HEAD ON OR SHELVE IT

In considering repair of a corneal laceration, it is important to evaluate the anatomy of the laceration and determine if the laceration is vertical (perpendicular) or oblique (shelved or beveled) (Figure 20-1). To understand the importance of this point, we must first consider several basic concepts about the cornea and its response to an incision or laceration.

- The normal cornea flattens over any vertical (perpendicular) incision. The cornea flattening effect from an incision or laceration is due to wound gape, similar to the effect seen with RK or arcuate keratotomy. This results in a longer arc length and, therefore, a longer radius of curvature. Clinically, this is seen on keratometry as corneal flattening. Additionally, this flattening effect increases as incisions approach the visual axis.
- The cornea flattens directly over any sutured incision. Traumatic lacerations are associated with even greater flattening when sutures are used to close the wound. This effect is exacerbated by longer sutures and persists in the postoperative period.
- Vertical (perpendicular) corneal lacerations gape more than shelved (beveled) corneal lacerations. This effect is referred to as the valve rule of Eisner. In practice, this means that vertical incisions (lacerations) tend to open spontaneously and require sutures, while shelved incisions (lacerations) may close spontaneously. It also means that because vertical incisions gape more, they are also associated with more cornea flattening and usually require more sutures to close the wound.

In understanding these principles and analyzing the physical properties of a corneal laceration, a structured surgical approach can be taken to repair the wound. In practice, this means that vertical (perpendicular) incisions should be closed first with good tissue coaptation. Shelved (beveled) incisions should be closed next, with fewer sutures and less tissue compression.

Always Remember…

Evaluate the anatomy of a corneal laceration to determine if it is vertical or shelved. Always release iris incarceration prior to suturing. If unsuccessful, place temporary sutures and release the incarceration on each side of the sutures before completing closure.

Figure 20-1 (Pearl 81). Vertical corneal incisions and lacerations gape and open spontaneously, while beveled incisions gape less and may close spontaneously. (Adapted from Shingleton BJ, Hersh PS, Kenyon KR, eds. *Eye Trauma*. St. Louis, MO: Mosby Year Book; 1991.)

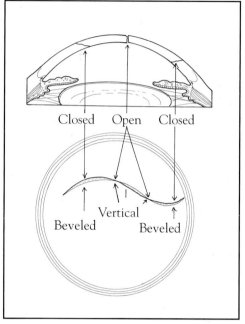

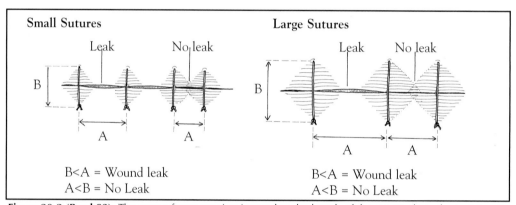

Figure 20-2 (Pearl 82). The zone of compression is equal to the length of the suture along the incision. To prevent wound leak, shorter sutures need to be closer together, while longer sutures can be spaced further apart. (Adapted from Shingleton BJ, Hersh PS, Kenyon KR, eds. *Eye Trauma*. St. Louis, MO: Mosby Year Book; 1991.)

PEARL #82: THE COMPRESSION FACTOR AND WOUND OVERRIDE

Most corneal lacerations require suturing because tissue compression is necessary to prevent wound leak and maintain tissue coaptation. An important concept in suture repair is the zone of compression (Figure 20-2). This is the amount of adjacent tissue compression along an incision or laceration where the suture is placed. Generally, the zone of compression produced by a suture is equal to the length of that suture. Therefore, assuming equal tightness, longer sutures produce a larger zone of compression, necessitating fewer sutures to close an incision (laceration) and keep it watertight. However, longer sutures also create more tissue distortion including astigmatism and increase the risk of tissue necrosis. Thus, longer sutures, while useful in closing traumatic corneal lacerations, should be avoided in the visual axis (Figure 20-3).

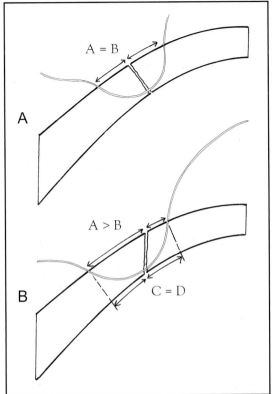

Figure 20-3 (Pearl 82). Corneal laceration repair. (A) Longer compression sutures are placed peripherally near the limbus. (B) Shorter appositional sutures are placed centrally to minimize flattening and restore sphericity. (Adapted from Shingleton BJ, Hersh PS, Kenyon KR, eds. *Eye Trauma.* St. Louis, MO: Mosby Year Book; 1991.)

One of the major issues when suturing the cornea for any reason is wound override. This is particularly a problem with traumatic corneal lacerations because tissue edema and ill-defined tissue edges often make corneal tissue coaptation especially challenging. Corneal wound and incision override produces an irregular corneal surface that disrupts epithelial wound healing. The resulting irregular corneal surface affects the precorneal tear film and visual quality. Furthermore, corneal wound override stimulates a microwedge resection, causing additional corneal flattening over the area of wedge resection and steepening of the involved meridian. Finally, incision override can lead to excess corneal scarring due to exposure of corneal stroma to the adjacent corneal epithelium.

Ideal suture placement in corneal incisions depends on the anatomy of the laceration. Different suture placement approaches are required for vertical (perpendicular) lacerations as opposed to oblique (shelved or beveled) lacerations.

For vertical corneal lacerations, the corneal sutures should be centered over the wound at 90% depth, so the suture entry site and the exit site are equidistant from the wound margins (Figure 20-4A). This will minimize corneal wound override and provide good tissue coaptation. If the suture entry site is shorter than the suture exit site, wound override will ensue. This happens because the longer suture exit site overlaps the short suture entry site when the suture is tightened.

Oblique corneal lacerations require a different approach. In this case, if the suture entry and exit sites are centered on the anterior aspect of the corneal laceration, tissue distortion and corneal wound override occur. To prevent this problem, placement of the corneal suture should be centered on the posterior aspect of the corneal laceration, not the anterior aspect as with vertical lacerations. This means that the suture entry and exit sites will be displaced with respect to the anterior portion of the corneal laceration (Figure 20-4B). Again, 90% tissue depth on both sides of the corneal wound is ideal. Using this technique, the result is a corneal wound repair with minimal tissue override and minimal induced astigmatism. Figures 20-5 and 20-6 show lacerations repaired according to the above guidelines.

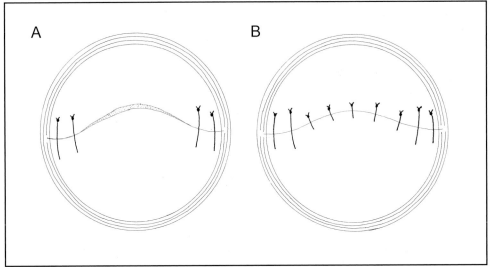

Figure 20-4 (Pearl 82). (A) In perpendicular incisions and lacerations, the suture must be placed equi-distant and equal depth (90%) to prevent tissue override. (B) In oblique incisions and lacerations, the suture should be centered over the posterior aspect of the wound and not over the anterior aspect as in perpendicular lacerations. (Adapted from Shingleton BJ, Hersh PS, Kenyon KR, eds. *Eye Trauma*. St. Louis, MO: Mosby Year Book; 1991.)

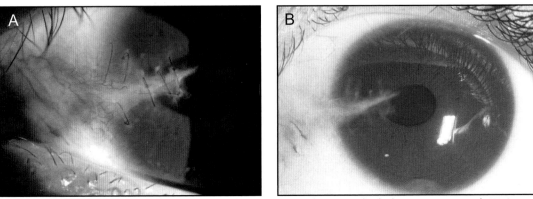

Figure 20-5 (Pearl 82). (A) Sutured corneal laceration illustrating the principles before suture removal. (B) Sutured corneal laceration illustrating the principles after suture removal.

Always Remember…

Vertical and oblique corneal lacerations require different suturing techniques. As opposed to surgical wounds, no two corneal lacerations are the same, but the principles of corneal laceration repair never change.

PEARL #83: THE SUTURELESS REPAIR OF CORNEAL LACERATIONS

Certainly, most corneal lacerations necessitate suturing, but occasionally, there are situations where suturing may not be required. As discussed previously, the length of a corneal laceration and incision is an important determination in corneal flattening and posttraumatic astigmatism. Therefore, longer cor-neal wounds should be closed in the manner described above. However, for small simple full-thickness corneal lacerations without evidence of other ocular tissue involvement, suturing may not be mandatory.

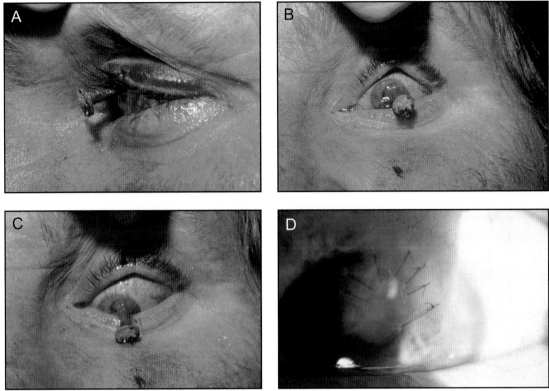

Figure 20-6 (Pearl 82). (A, B, C) Nail gun injury. (D) Corneal laceration repair after nail gun injury. (Courtesy of Dimitri T. Azar, MD and Jonathan Primack, MD, Massachusetts Eye and Ear Infirmary.)

One may consider not suturing corneal lacerations that satisfy the following five requirements:
- The laceration length is 3 mm or less.
- There is no intraocular tissue to the wound.
- There are no other ocular structures involved.
- There is no foreign material in the laceration (organic or otherwise).
- The wound is a self-sealing or Seidel positive only with provocation.

In addition to the length of the corneal laceration, the wound should not be nondisplaced, beveled, and/or edematous. This will help to maintain a watertight wound. If the criteria are met, then a bandage contact lens should be placed over the cornea. Our preference is a thick, large diameter contact lens such as a Plano T (Bausch & Lomb Surgical, St. Louis, Mo) or Permalens (CooperVision, Fairport, NY). This lens should be left in place for about 3 weeks. Antibiotic and steroid drops can be safely given with the contact lens in place.

An aqueous suppressant can be used to minimize wound leaking acutely. We discourage the use of bromonidine because it can dry the ocular surface and make the contact lens uncomfortable. Pressure patching can also be considered in conjunction with the contact lens acutely.

Using this method to treat corneal lacerations requires a very cooperative adult patient. We do not recommend this treatment management for children and strongly advise suturing all corneal lacerations in children.

Always Remember...

Most corneal lacerations require suturing; however, for small simple corneal lacerations, if certain criteria are met, no suturing may be required.

Bibliography

Barr CC. Prognostic factors in corneoscleral lacerations. *Arch Ophthalmol.* 1983;101:919-924.

Eagling EM. Perforating injuries of the eye. *Br J Ophthalmol.* 1976;60:732-736.

Eisner G. *Eye Surgery: An Introduction to Operative Techniques.* New York, NY: Springer Verlag; 1980:37.

Rowsey JJ. Ten caveats in keratorefractive surgery. *Ophthalmology.* 1983;90:148-155.

Rowsey JJ, Hays JC. Refractive reconstruction for acute eye injuries. *Ophthalmic Surg.* 1984;15:569-574.

CHAPTER 21

THREE
PEARLS IN SUCCESSFUL APPLICATION OF CYANOACRYLATE GLUE TO THE CORNEA

Jonathan D. Primack, MD

Ophthalmologic indications for applying cyanoacrylate glue to the anterior segment of the eye (not US FDA approved) include corneal ulceration with progressive thinning, descemetocele, and small corneal perforations (usually <2 mm). Infection is the most common cause of corneal thinning and perforation, but similar conditions may arise from a variety of etiologies including inflammation, ocular surface disease, and trauma. Following glue application, it is important to recognize and treat the patient's underlying problem with the appropriate therapeutic modality (ie, antibiotics, antivirals, immunosuppression, lubrication, etc) in order to arrest the disease process.

PEARL #84: INDICATIONS: TO GLUE OR NOT TO GLUE?

The glue covering ulcerated or perforated tissue provides immediate and long-term benefits. In cases of progressive ulceration or descemetocele formation, the glue functions as a covering for the nonepithelialized, thinning stroma. Exposed stroma may be susceptible to inflammatory reactions that release enzymes responsible for corneal degradation. Glue presumably acts as a barrier to neutrophil migration and protects against further thinning. This may arrest keratolysis and prevent a nonhealing ulcer from progressing to a descemetocele or the latter from becoming a frank perforation. Clinicians should not hesitate to apply glue early in cases of mild to moderate thinning because waiting may result in further corneal decompensation. In a perforated globe, the glue provides a watertight barrier, preventing infection and restoring ocular integrity. This may allow reparative surgical procedures such as penetrating keratoplasty to be postponed until the eye is less inflamed and more likely to experience improved surgical outcomes.

Adhesive should not be applied in thinned areas covered by epithelium. Glue protects melting, ulcerated stromal tissue. If a thinned area is not ulcerated (ie, epithelium is intact), the glue serves no purpose because the tissue is already covered. Epithelialized corneas rarely experience stromal thinning. If it does occur, it is usually from noninflammatory conditions such as Terrien's marginal degeneration, keratoconus, pellucid marginal degeneration, furrow degeneration, or dellen.

In approximately one-third of cases, the glue induces a healing response that precludes the need for surgery. Ideally, as an ulcer heals, epithelium will grow under the glue and spontaneously dislodge it, revealing intact tissue. In perforations, the tissue underlying the glue may experience collagen deposition and scar formation. If epithelium grows to cover the scar, the adhesive will slough. Figure 21-1A illustrates a peripheral corneal melt and perforation secondary to keratoconjunctivitis sicca in a patient with autoimmune disease (note the pupil peaking toward the perforation). This patient was treated with cyanoacrylate glue (Figure 21-1B), which extruded several months after its initial application. Examination at that time (Figure 21-1C) demonstrated a fully epithelialized, healed corneal scar with blood vessels traversing the once perforated stroma. Figure 21-2 illustrates another example of a perforated peripheral corneal ulcer that healed successfully with cyanoacrylate glue. Figure 21-3 shows glue applied to peripheral ulcerative keratitis (PUK).

Always Remember…

Do not wait for a persistent corneal ulcer to result in severe stromal tissue loss before applying glue.

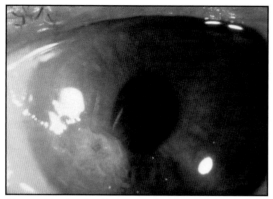

Figure 21-1A (Pearl 84). A peripheral corneal melt and perforation secondary to keratoconjunctivitis sicca in a patient with autoimmune disease. (Courtesy of Deborah P. Langston, MD, Massachusetts Eye and Ear Infirmary.)

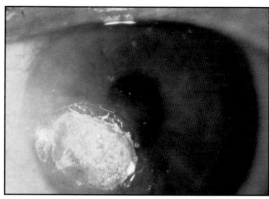

Figure 21-1B (Pearl 84). Cyanoacrylate glue applied to the above lesion. (Courtesy of Deborah P. Langston, MD, Massachusetts Eye and Ear Infirmary.)

Figure 21-1C (Pearl 84). A fully epithelialized, healed corneal scar with blood vessels traversing the once perforated stroma is the result after successful cyanoacrylate glue application. (Courtesy of Deborah P. Langston, MD, Massachusetts Eye and Ear Infirmary.)

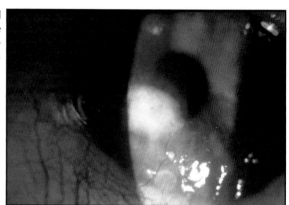

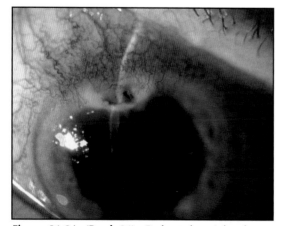

Figure 21-2A (Pearl 84). Perforated peripheral corneal ulcer in a patient with underlying autoimmune disease. (Courtesy of Jonathan Primack, MD, North Shore-Long Island Jewish Medical Center Department of Ophthalmology.)

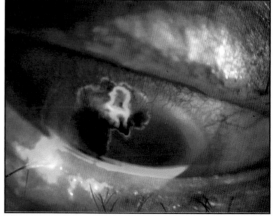

Figure 21-2B (Pearl 84). Fluorescein is applied to ulcer to perform a Seidel test. (Courtesy of Jonathan Primack, MD, North Shore-Long Island Jewish Medical Center Department of Ophthalmology.)

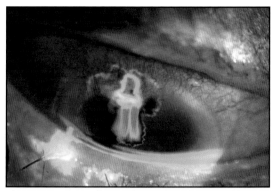

Figure 21-2C (Pearl 84). The egress of aqueous humor with its waterfall appearance confirms that the ulcer has perforated. (Courtesy of Jonathan Primack, MD, North Shore-Long Island Jewish Medical Center Department of Ophthalmology.)

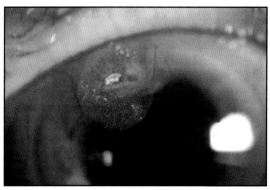

Figure 21-2D (Pearl 84). After obtaining the appropriate cultures and slides, cyanoacrylate glue is applied on a 2 mm plastic disc and placed over the perforated ulcer. The ulceration is successfully sealed. (Courtesy of Jonathan Primack, MD, North Shore-Long Island Jewish Medical Center Department of Ophthalmology.)

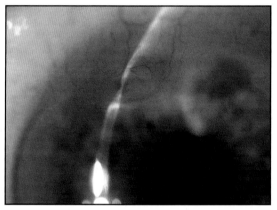

Figure 21-2E (Pearl 84). Same patient several months later. The glue has spontaneously dislodged, revealing a well-vascularized thin layer of scar tissue. (Courtesy of Jonathan Primack, MD, North Shore-Long Island Jewish Medical Center Department of Ophthalmology.)

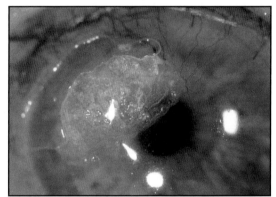

Figure 21-3 (Pearl 84). Cyanoacrylate glue applied to PUK.

PEARL #85: GLUING TIPS AND AVOIDING STICKY SITUATIONS

The commercially available forms of cyanoacrylate glue differ from one another by the length of their carbon side chains. Unfortunately, those with the greatest bonding strength are the least clinically tolerated. Medical grade isobutyl-2-cyanoacrylate (4 carbon side chain) has excellent adhesive properties and negligible, deleterious side effects. It is currently the glue of choice for ophthalmic indications. Store-bought "super glue" (methyl-2-cyanoacrylate [1 carbon side chain]) can cause irritation secondary to formaldehyde liberated into the tear film during normal polymer degradation. It is not recommended for ophthalmic use but is commonly used in economically strained areas.

Glue can be applied while the patient is sitting upright at the slit lamp or is lying supine under the microscope. The former is preferred when gluing ulcers and the latter is good for perforations given the beneficial effect of gravity. The physician may wish to prep and drape the involved eye before gluing; however, a sterile environment is not necessary, and these procedures are often performed in examining rooms. Once positioned, topical anesthesia is administered in both eyes, and a speculum is placed between the eyelids. Loose or necrotic tissue should be removed because glue adhering to such material may easily become dislodged. Cultures may be taken at this point if there is concern of infection.

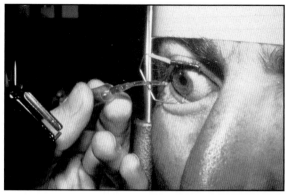

Figure 21-4 (Pearl 85). Application of glue to the cornea at the slit-lamp biomicroscope. (Reprinted with permission of Albert DM, Jakobiec FA. *Principles and Practice of Ophthalmology*. Philadelphia, PA: WB Saunders Company; 1994:230.)

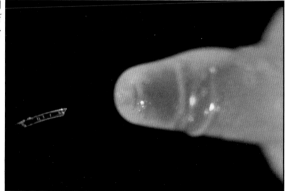

Figure 21-5 (Pearl 85). A micropipette may be used to remove the glue from its container. (Courtesy of Claes H. Dohlman, MD, Massachusetts Eye and Ear Infirmary.)

Vitreous or foreign contaminants should be carefully extracted from the perforation site. If the iris has prolapsed into the wound, one may consider gently injecting filtered air or a viscoelastic agent through either the perforation or a paracentesis site to gently move it aside and prevent its incorporation into the glue. Viscoelastic agents can raise the IOP, so use sparingly. Prior to application, it is extremely important to remove the surrounding 1 to 2 mm of epithelium and to thoroughly dry the stromal bed. The latter may be difficult in a perforation with a steady egress of aqueous humor. Multiple cellulose spears can be used to successively dry the surface before glue is applied. If this technique proves difficult, one may very carefully place pressure on the anterior segment to express a bolus of aqueous. This may provide a window of opportunity to dry the surface and seal the perforation.

All corneal gluing techniques share one common goal: Plug the perforation or cover the ulceration with the smallest amount of glue possible. Excess adhesive on the ocular surface can cause irritation, limit the clinician's view, mask progressive disease, and result in early displacement of the glue.

Multiple techniques of cyanoacrylate glue application have been described. If provided in an applicator, the glue may be applied directly to the cornea (Figure 21-4). Alternatively, one may use a micropipette to remove the glue from its container (Figure 21-5) and apply it to the desired location in a controlled fashion (Figure 21-6). A cellulose spear also functions well if gluing a thinned ulcer. It absorbs a negligible amount of adhesive and spreads a fine coat of glue over the defect. Other methods include using a 27-gauge needle (tapping the top with your fingertip will deliver a drop of glue at the beveled end), the blunt end of a cellulose spear, or the broken-off end of a cotton-tipped applicator. One may also use a 2 to 3 mm polyethylene disc attached by a drop of ointment to the end of a wooden applicator stick (author's preferred technique). Glue is applied to the disc's undersurface then held against the perforation site for approximately 30 seconds. The applicator stick is withdrawn, leaving the disc in place with the glue.

Even when glue is placed in an appropriate fashion, it is not uncommon for it to dislodge and require more than one application. Figure 21-7 is an example of excessive corneal glue. Under such

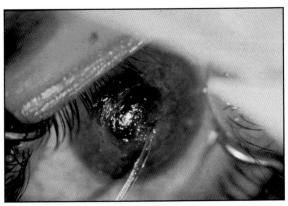

Figure 21-6 (Pearl 85). Application of glue to the cornea with a micropipette. (Courtesy of Claes H. Dohlman, MD, Massachusetts Eye and Ear Infirmary.)

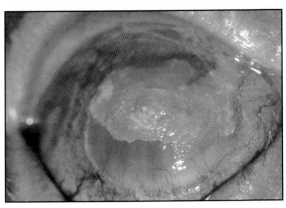

Figure 21-7 (Pearl 85). Excessive amounts of cyanoacrylate glue to the cornea. (Courtesy of Claes H. Dohlman, MD, Massachusetts Eye and Ear Infirmary.)

circumstances, the glue can be gently removed using a jeweler's forceps and the process started again. Caution should be exercised, however, when removing glue from descemetoceles, as even mild manipulation may result in perforation.

The above procedural variations are possible because glue polymerization does not occur on or inside the delivering instrument. The glue only hardens once in the presence of anions such as OH–, which is abundant in water or aqueous. The physician may use this property to his or her advantage and hasten polymerization by applying basic salt solution to the glue after proper placement on the cornea.

Perforations larger than 2 mm present a challenge. Ideally, one wishes to close the perforation and avoid surgery, but glue can only efficiently seal a small area. Complications reported when gluing large perforations include inadvertent entry into the anterior chamber, leading to corneal decompensation or cataract. Cases have occurred requiring surgical removal of intraocular glue. Several techniques have been devised to avoid these pitfalls. A partial thickness corneal or scleral patch can be fashioned and glued over a descemetocele or perforation. Another clever technique first used by Droutsas involves crisscrossing the perforation site with a running 10-0 nylon suture (Figure 21-8). This provides scaffolding upon which the glue may polymerize and seal the perforation.

Always Remember…

Use medical grade cyanoacrylate adhesive to limit ocular surface toxicity.

Scrape the corneal epithelium and dry the ocular surface with a microsponge before placing the glue.

Use the least amount of glue needed to cover the ulcer or seal the perforation.

Larger perforations (>2 mm) may be closed using glue applied over a scaffold of 10-0 nylon suture.

Figure 21-8 (Pearl 85). 10-0 nylon sutures can be used as scaffolding to glue corneal perforations larger than 2 mm in surface area.

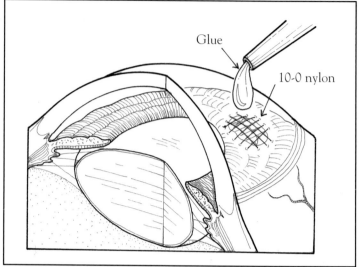

PEARL #86: MAINTENANCE OF GLUE ON THE OCULAR SURFACE

Proper management after cyanoacrylate glue placement will help prevent potential complications. Once the glue is in place, the site should be examined to ensure the entire ulcer or perforation is adequately covered. A Seidel test is helpful in the latter. If positive, further gluing is indicated until the opening is sealed. A therapeutic high-water-content soft contact lens such as a Permalens or Kontur is then placed to prevent the mechanical forces of the eyelids from dislodging the glue. This step also decreases foreign body sensation. The patient should be re-examined 30 minutes after gluing to check that the adhesive is in place and that the anterior chamber has reformed. Aqueous suppressants should be prescribed in patients with perforations to limit the stress on the glue. Topical lubrication and punctal plugs may benefit dry eye patients. All patients should be given a protective shield because minimal trauma may loosen the glue.

Patients receiving corneal glue are at an increased risk for infection. Indeed, some patients may have a concurrent corneal infection at the time of glue application. The antibacterial effect of cyanoacrylate adhesive is questionable, and all patients who receive glue and a bandage contact lens for a sterile ulcer should receive topical antibiotics at least 3 times a day to serve as prophylaxis against bacterial keratitis. Infections have been documented to occur under intact glue, so patients must be monitored carefully. Physicians may wish to prescribe oral fluoroquinolones for individuals with a history of perforation given their high ocular tissue concentrations. Infected corneal perforations are treated with fortified topical and IV antibiotics. Slides and culture results should guide the choice of therapeutic agents. A consult by a retina specialist is recommended if there is a concern of endophthalmitis.

Initially, postadhesive placement patients should be seen frequently. It is preferable to move the contact lens aside with a cotton tip applicator at the slit lamp rather than removing it (Figure 21-9). Removal of the contact lens to examine the patient can lead to both lens contamination and displacement of the glue.

Always Remember...

Perform a Seidel test after applying adhesive to the perforated cornea.

Use topical antibiotics to prevent bandage contact lens-related infections.

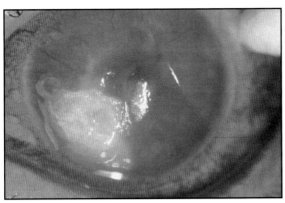

Figure 21-9 (Pearl 86). It is preferable to move a bandage contact lens aside with a cotton tip applicator at the slit lamp rather than removing it. (Courtesy of Deborah P. Langston, MD, Massachusetts Eye and Ear Infirmary.)

Bibliography

Cavanaugh TB, Gottsch JD. Infectious keratitis and cyanoacrylate adhesive. *Am J Ophthalmol.* 1991;111:466-472.

Eiferman RA, Snyder JW. Antibacterial effect of cyanoacrylate glue. *Arch Ophthalmol.* 1983;101:958-960.

Erday RA, Lindahl RJ, Temnycky GO, et al. Technique for application of tissue adhesive for corneal perforations. *Ophthal Surg.* 1991;22:352-354.

Honig MA, Rapuano CJ. Management of corneal perforations. In: Krachmer JH, Mannis MJ, Holland EJ, eds. *Cornea: Surgery of the Cornea and Conjunctiva.* Boston, MA: Mosby;1997:1818-1825.

Leahey AB, Gottsch JD, Stark WJ. Clinical experience with n-butyl cyanoacrylate (nexacryl) tissue adhesive. *Ophthalmology.* 1993;100:173-180.

Moschos M, Droutsas D, Boussalis P, Tsioulias G. Clinical experience with cyanoacrylate tissue adhesive. *Doc Ophthalmol.* 1997;93:237-245.

Refojo MF, Dohlman CH, Koliopoulos J. Adhesives in ophthalmology: a review. *Surv Ophthalmol.* 1971;15(4):217-236.

CHAPTER 22

SIX PEARLS
IN CHALLENGING CORNEAL SURGERY

Esen K. Akpek, MD; Rana Altan-Yaycioglu, MD; and Walter J. Stark, MD

Vision-impairing corneal disease is second only to cataract as the leading cause of global blindness, affecting nearly 10 million people around the world. Fortunately, great progress has been made in recent years in both the medical and surgical aspects of managing corneal diseases. In this chapter, we address some of the challenging corneal disorders. Emphasis is placed on the practical aspects of the management.

PEARL #87: THE NEUROTROPHIC CORNEA

The etiology of the neurotrophic cornea varies considerably. Damage to the trigeminal nerve may result from surgery or trauma (eg, rhizotomy for trigeminal neuralgia, cerebrovascular accident, aneurysms), tumors (eg, neurofibroma or angioma), or infections (eg, herpes zoster ophthalmicus or herpes simplex keratitis). The trigeminal nerve acts as the afferent branch for reflex tear production. Its dysfunction results in decreased lacrimal and conjunctival tear secretion as well as poor epithelial adhesion owing to the impaired attachment complex formation in the basement membrane of the corneal epithelium.

In many patients with acquired or congenital corneal hypoesthesia (or anesthesia), the cornea may appear normal at first or exhibit only mild punctate epithelial erosions. However, because of the thinning of the epithelium from a reduction in neurotrophic stimuli and poor adhesion, recurrent erosions will occur with minor trauma or spontaneously. Once an epithelial defect develops, infection or stromal ulceration often will follow due to the difficulty in re-epithelialization. Aggressive use of topical preservative-free lubricants along with high water content bandage contact lenses is the first line of treatment in clean epithelial defects. Autologous serum treatment also seems promising for the restoration of the ocular surface epithelial integrity, particularly in patients with a sicca syndrome. Nerve growth factor has been proposed as an important component of wound healing and tissue repair process in vivo and in vitro. Nerve growth factor is a neurotrophic and immunomodulatory factor, contributing to the control of cutaneous morphogenesis, wound healing, and inflammatory responses. Recently, topical administration of nerve growth factor was shown to accelerate the rate of wound healing in clinical studies.

Punctal plugs or cauterization of the puncti is also used to preserve the tear film bathing the ocular surface.

Mediolateral tarsorrhaphy should be considered in patients with incomplete blink or lagophthalmos who have persistent epithelial defects with an associated stromal ulceration (Figure 22-1).

If the ulcer progresses, application of tissue adhesives should be considered as the first line of treatment in impending or small perforations, particularly in inflamed corneas, due to their additional inhibitory effect on polymorph nuclear leukocyte migration (Figure 22-2) (see Chapter 21).

A lamellar corneal graft may be considered if the glue application fails with further stromal thinning or if the area of the thinning is of considerable size. Conjunctival flap is usually considered as the last resort in patients with recurrent corneal melting. A relatively new surgical method is to transplant a multilayer cryopreserved human amniotic membrane over the neurotrophic ulcer for ocular surface reconstruction (see also Chapter 19).

Figure 22-1 (Pearl 87). Healed corneal surface with stromal scarring following a permanent mediolateral tarsorrhaphy in a patient with neurotrophic keratitis and lagophthalmos due to herpes zoster.

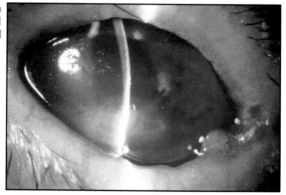

Figure 22-2 (Pearl 87). Application of tissue adhesive with a 21-gauge needle for a small central corneal perforation due to trauma.

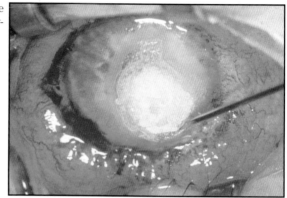

Figure 22-3 (Pearl 87). Cauterization of lower puncti in a patient with significant surface desiccation and recurrent epithelial defects following fifth nerve ablation due to trigeminal neuralgia.

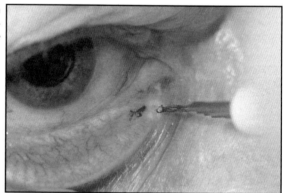

Always Remember...

Always use prophylactic topical antibiotic and cycloplegic eye drops along with bandage contact lenses, since secondary infections and sterile hypopyon are common in neurotrophic corneas.

Anesthetic eyes are at higher risk of graft failure. Therefore, corneal sensation should be assessed preoperatively to appropriately select patients for successful future transplantation.

Penetrating keratoplasty in an anesthetic corneal bed has a poor success rate and, thus, should be approached with caution. Mediolateral tarsorrhaphy with or without occlusion/cauterization of lacrimal puncti should always be performed at the time of corneal surgery to reduce surface desiccation (Figure 22-3).

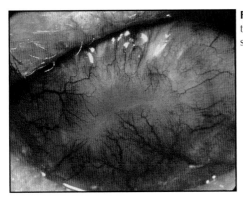

Figure 22-4 (Pearl 88). Corneal surgery should be deferred until the neovessels regress with time and topical steroid treatment in such a heavily vascularized eye.

Keratoprosthesis can be recommended in eyes with significantly poor ocular surface disease. However, postoperative glaucoma is considerable.

Pearl #88: The Vascularized Cornea

If corneal surgery is contemplated, it is best to plan ahead and use moderate doses of topical steroids for several weeks before the corneal surgery to suppress the neovascularization (Figure 22-4). Yellow dye laser to close down the vascular channels will only work temporarily. Any structural abnormalities causing or promoting the neovascularization, such as lagophthalmos, trichiasis, or keratinization of lid margins, should be addressed before the corneal surgery. Performing a penetrating keratoplasty in a vascularized corneal bed may be challenging due to excessive bleeding. Topical application of chilled epinephrine (1:1000) to constrict the vessels and tamponading with viscoelastic can be useful to manage excessive bleeding.

In glaucomatous eyes, meticulous control of IOP before keratoplasty is mandatory. Surgical techniques that may help to decrease the risk of postoperative glaucoma are oversized grafts in aphakic or pseudophakic grafts, lysis of previous anterior synechiae, well sutured wound to prevent a postoperative flat chamber and synechiae formation, and simultaneous trabeculectomy in poorly controlled glaucoma. If these methods fail, cyclocryotherapy and tube shunt implants should be considered.

Always Remember…

The immunologic rejection capacity of a vascularized recipient bed is considerably higher than otherwise. Hourly use of topical steroids along with topical cyclosporine for several months in the postoperative period may be needed to prevent an allograft rejection.

Asymmetric neovascularization may cause local contraction of the wound and loosening of sutures, which can result in irritation, infection, or rejection of the transplant. Therefore, interrupted sutures are preferable because these may be removed selectively.

Pearl #89: Enhancing Regrafting Success

Every year, approximately 42,000 corneal transplants are performed in the United States. Although penetrating keratoplasty is successful in more than 90% of cases, a considerable proportion of grafts fail (Figure 22-5A and 22-5B) depending chiefly on the recipient's corneal disease, such as aphakic bullous keratopathy, or the presence of preoperative peripheral anterior synechiae, need for intraoperative anterior vitrectomy, and neovascularization of the recipient cornea. Immune-mediated rejection is the leading cause of graft failure. Unfortunately, the incidence of rejection is higher and the level of visual rehabilitation attained is less effective following regrafting than primary surgery. Therefore, a rigorous preoperative evaluation to address preexisting adverse conditions and meticulous patient education

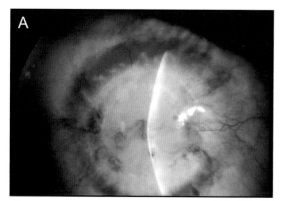

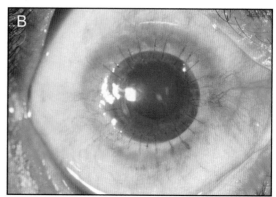

Figure 22-5 (Pearl 89). The Boston Keratoprosthesis type I.

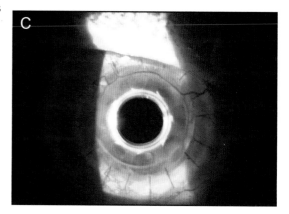

regarding symptoms of graft rejection are of paramount importance. Patients should be instructed to inform their doctor immediately if they encounter light sensitivity, decrease in visual acuity, discomfort, and/or redness in their eyes. A useful mnemonic for patients to remember the warning signs of rejection is RSVP (redness, sensitivity to light, vision change, pain). The Boston keratoprosthesis developed by Claes Dohlman, MD is emerging as a reliable alternative in cases with multiple graft failures (Figure 22-5C).

Eyes repeatedly subjected to operative procedures are more likely to develop other problems such as cataract, raised IOP, retinal detachment, or cystoid macular edema. Always exclude other possible causes of decrease in visual acuity before considering regrafting.

Always cut the donor button before removing the recipient's cornea. The size of the graft is determined before the surgery and is generally the same size as the previous graft used. In cases with previous grafts larger than 8.0 mm, a graft of 8.0 or less in diameter is preferred because of the increasing risk of rejection with increasing diameter of transplants.

Most donor buttons are 7.5 to 8.0 mm in diameter and 0.5 mm oversized, except in keratoconus, where use of 0.25 mm oversized or same-sized graft helps to reduce postoperative myopia. However, cauterization of the central host cornea prior to trephination will result in contraction; therefore, a 0.5 mm larger graft can be used.

Anterior synechiae, if present, must be cut with Vannas scissors. Viscodissection can be tried at the iridocorneal angle to break goniosynechia.

During a rejection episode, do not hesitate to treat with topical steroids. The recommended dose is prednisolone acetate every hour while awake. Even if the patient is a steroid responder, treat with potent topical steroids until IOP increases. Reduce the inflammation as quickly as possible, and treat the pressure rise as it occurs. Switch to weaker steroids or discontinue only if IOP cannot be medically controlled and if there is significant risk of damage to the optic nerve.

Always Remember…

If the previous surgery was performed within less than 1 year, grasping the donor cornea with a forceps inserted through an incision at the host-recipient junction, unless there is significant neovascularization, can often easily unzip the donor graft.

The chances of rejection are directly proportional with the number of quadrants of neovascularization and the number of previous rejections.

Sometimes, endothelial rejection may not be associated with keratic precipitates and ciliary injection. Therefore, it is useful to measure the corneal thickness objectively with pachymeter. Always consider early rejection if 10% increase in corneal thickness is observed, and treat with steroids. It is remarkable to see how many of these corneas get thinner and clearer with the topical steroid treatment.

PEARL #90: EPITHELIAL DOWNGROWTH

Wound leakage, ocular hypotony, and loss of blood-aqueous barrier may predispose to invasion of conjunctival or corneal epithelial cells into the anterior chamber. The proliferating cells lead to corneal endothelial decompensation, glaucoma, and eventually phthisis. Owing to the considerable advances in microsurgical techniques and materials, epithelial downgrowth into the eye following intraocular surgery or trauma is rare. The key to successfully managing these cases is early diagnosis. Once the epithelial ingrowth is widespread, prognosis is poor because the extensive destructive therapy often destroys the eye as well as the invading epithelial tissue.

Diagnosis can be made by slit lamp examination. Confocal microscopy is a newer method that allows noninvasive in vivo examination of the cornea.

Epithelial downgrowth should be distinguished from a fibrous retrocorneal membrane or an endothelial rejection line in cases of corneal grafts. Epithelial downgrowth is generally composed of a single layer of epithelial cells, but the advancing edge is multilayered and clinically appears thickened and scalloped.

To test the extent of epithelial invasion onto the iris surface, laser photocoagulation with a spot size of 200 to 500 µm and 0.1 to 0.5 seconds is placed on the iris. If no epithelial cells are present, the burns turn dark and simply contract. If the burned surface turns white, it indicates epithelial invasion. Lasering may also serve as a treatment, particularly in the early cases. Once the extent of epithelial downgrowth has been identified, involved iris tissue can be removed through a three-port vitrectomy approach. A straight transvitreal cryoprobe is then used to destruct the retrocorneal cells directly. The retrocorneal cells can sometimes be peeled in sheets using intraocular forceps. However, it is still necessary to freeze the bed to prevent recurrences.

Intracameral 5 fluorouracil application following the viscodissection of the membrane and peeling from the corneal endothelium was reported to be effective.

Always Remember…

In eyes with epithelial downgrowth confined to the cornea, transcorneal freezing with a regular cryoprobe may be sufficient, especially if the area affected is small. An intracameral air bubble is useful to provide an insulating effect and a more effective, controlled destruction. In more advanced cases intracameral 5-FU can be applied.

PEARL #91: CONTRALATERAL CORNEAS IN MONOCULAR PATIENTS (AUTOKERATOPLASTY)

Autokeratoplasty can be considered in monocular patients with a clear cornea in the fellow eye. The blind eye's cornea is used as donor material. The advantage is the elimination of the possibility of an allograft rejection. However, the endothelial cell loss and continuous decrease in the endothelial cell density in the postoperative period is comparable to allografts and can be minimized by topical corticosteroids. The basic surgical principles of penetrating keratoplasty apply to autokeratoplasty. However, because the rejection is not a problem, a larger graft may be preferred for optical purposes. Ipsilateral rotational autokeratoplasty can also be considered as an alternative procedure to penetrating keratoplasty.

Surgical technique is not straightforward. The first step is to trim the cadaveric donor cornea. Its diameter should be 1 mm larger than the intended graft size (eg, if an 8.0-mm graft is desired, the cadaveric donor cornea should be trimmed 9 mm in diameter). Then the patient's donor cornea is cut (8.5 mm in this case) and transferred into a moist chamber. The patient's donor eye is closed with the cadaveric donor cornea. Attention is then directed to the patient's recipient eye. The opaque cornea of the recipient eye is trephined (8.0 mm). Then, the autograft (8.5 mm) is sutured onto the patient's recipient eye.

Always Remember...

Because graft rejection is not a concern in autokeratoplasty, a larger graft is preferred for optical purposes.

Limited postoperative topical steroid use is sufficient since there is no risk of rejection.

PEARL #92: LAMELLAR KERATOPLASTY

Lamellar keratoplasty accounts for less than 1% of all corneal graft surgeries. Lamellar keratoplasty may be performed for optical purposes, although it is more frequently preferred for tectonic purposes for localized stromal thinning or perforation due to infectious diseases, trauma, or systemic collagen vascular diseases (Figures 22-6 and 22-7). As in the case of penetrating keratoplasty, the condition of the ocular surface is of utmost importance. Patients with exposure keratopathy, anesthetic cornea, or dry eyes will have a guarded prognosis. Lamellar keratoplasty should be approached with caution in eyes with active infectious keratitis or inflammation.

Donor tissue requirements are less stringent than in penetrating keratoplasty, thus, allowing the use of whole globe preservation in a moist chamber at 4°C for up to 2 weeks or, alternatively, cryopreservation or lyophilization.

Unlike the penetrating keratoplasty, the donor tissue is prepared once the recipient bed has been dissected. The graft should be the same thickness as the recipient bed and generally oversized in diameter by 0.5 mm. If the graft involves the limbus, a same-size graft is preferable. After the desired area for excision has been defined, the host cornea is trephined with a Hessburg-Barron or a hand-held trephine. A dissecting spatula (Martinez or cyclodialysis spatula or a Tooke or Paufique blade [Bausch & Lomb Surgical, St. Louis, Mo]) is introduced into the lips of the wound, and a lamellar dissection parallel to the corneal curvature is performed (Figure 22-8). If the lamellar keratoplasty is being performed for a corneal ectatic disorder, a paracentesis should be performed prior to suturing the graft to lower the IOP and flatten the anterior chamber to better allow flattening of the cornea (see Figure 22-8).

Once the lamellar keratectomy is complete, dissection of the graft can begin. If a whole globe is used, it is grasped with a 2 x 2 inch gauze sponge and wrapped along the equator of the globe. A small incision is made at the limbus, and the entire cornea is dissected to the desired depth with a dissecting spatula from limbus to limbus. The desired trephine is used to cut the desired size of lamellar graft, which is then transferred to the recipient bed. If a corneoscleral button is available, first the appropriate size of trephination is created, then the button is grasped with toothed forceps in two locations while Vannas scissors are used to trim the peripheral donor button (1 to 3 mm) from the endothelial side (Figure 22-9). A dry microsponge is initially used to remove the endothelial cell layer. It is usually quite difficult to remove DM, which is, therefore, left undisturbed.

In the postoperative period, topical steroids and antibiotics should be used at moderate doses for several weeks. Risk of local allograft rejection reaction is much less in the absence of endothelial transfer, and the visual consequences of stromal rejection tend to be less devastating than an endothelial

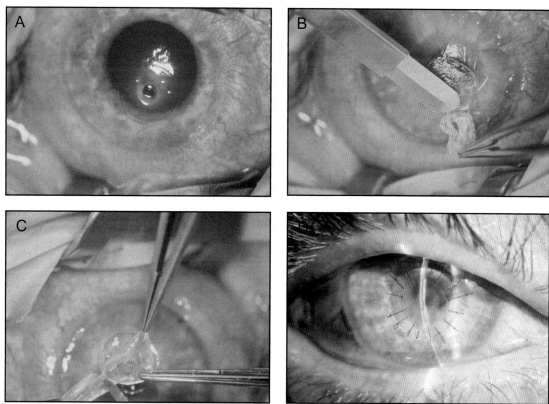

Figure 22-6 (Pearl 92). (A) Performing a lamellar keratoplasty in an eye with a small central perforation. The size of the recipient bed has been measured and marked with a hand-held trephine. (B) Preparing the recipient bed by lamellar keratectomy. (C) Dissection of the lamellar graft. (D) Postoperative 2-month appearance of the eye.

rejection. However, appropriate immunosuppression is essential in the presence of systemic collagen vascular diseases in order to prevent recurrent corneal melting and perforation.

The major source of visual loss and slow visual improvement in lamellar keratoplasty is the opacification and vascularization of the interface between the donor and host cornea. This is mainly due to the irregularities in the interface when the lamellar dissection is performed manually. Particularly, in cases where the lamellar keratoplasty is performed for optical purposes (ie, anterior stromal dystrophies, postinfectious scars, etc), the use of an automated microkeratome or the femtosecond intrastromal laser may yield better results.

Always Remember...

It is preferable to use tissue glue as the first line procedure to seal an impending or small perforation rather than a lamellar keratoplasty in corneas with active infection/inflammation.

Intrastromal viscoelastic, saline, air, or balanced salt solution may be used to facilitate intralamellar manual dissection.

The most serious complication of lamellar keratoplasty is accidental perforation during the lamellar keratectomy. This may be avoided by performing a paracentesis and reforming the anterior chamber with viscoelastic prior to dissection in order to increase the resistance of the globe.

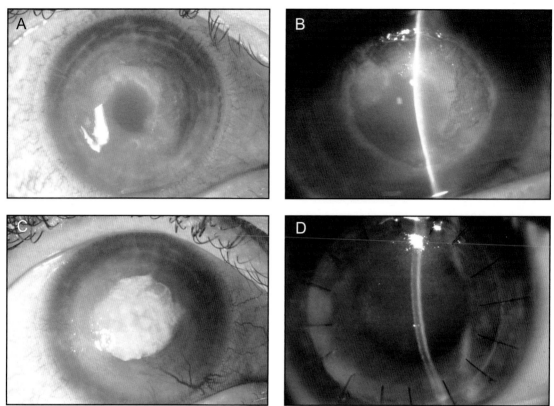

Figure 22-7 (Pearl 92). (A) Acanthamoeba keratitis: acute ring infiltrate; preoperative photo. (B) Acanthamoeba keratitis: fulminant infection; preoperative photo. (C) Acanthamoeba keratitis: vascularization, lipid deposition, and scarring 4 months postinfection. (D) Acanthamoeba keratitis: postlamellar keratoplasty. (Courtesy of the Massachusetts Eye and Ear Infirmary.)

Always Remember…

Have a tissue adhesive available for the repair of possible small perforations.

Fresh tissue should be made available in case of a wide perforation necessitating penetrating keratoplasty.

Wound leakage, ocular hypotony, and loss of blood-aqueous barrier may predispose to invasion of conjunctival or corneal epithelial cells into the anterior chamber. The proliferating cells lead to corneal endothelial decompensation, glaucoma, and eventually phthisis. Owing to the considerable advances in microsurgical techniques and materials, epithelial downgrowth into the eye following intraocular surgery or trauma is rare. The key to successfully managing these cases is early diagnosis. Once the epithelial ingrowth is widespread, prognosis is poor because the extensive destructive therapy often destroys the eye as well as the invading epithelial tissue.

Diagnosis can be made by slit lamp examination. Confocal microscopy is a newer method that allows noninvasive in vivo examination of the cornea.

Epithelial downgrowth should be distinguished from a fibrous retrocorneal membrane or an endothelial rejection line in cases of corneal grafts. Epithelial downgrowth is generally composed of a single layer of epithelial cells, but the advancing edge is multilayered and clinically appears thickened and scalloped.

To test the extent of epithelial invasion onto the iris surface, laser photocoagulation with a spot size of 200 to 500 mm and 0.1 to 0.5 seconds is placed on the iris. If no epithelial cells are present, the burns

Figure 22-8 (Pearl 92). Lamellar keratoplasty: a dissecting spatula (Martinez or cyclodialysis spatula or a Tooke or Paufique blade) is introduced into the lips of the wound, and a lamellar dissection parallel to the corneal curvature is performed on a dry stromal bed. If the lamellar keratoplasty is being performed for a corneal ectatic disorder, a paracentesis should be performed prior to suturing the graft to lower the IOP to better allow flattening of the cornea.

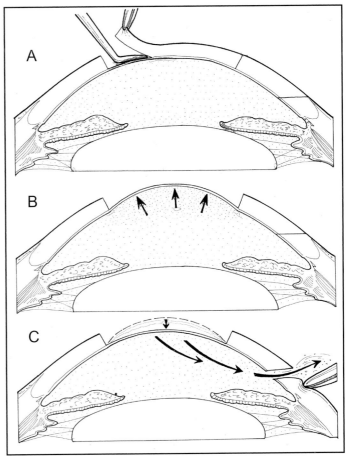

Figure 22-9 (Pearl 92). Lamellar keratoplasty: a dry microsponge is initially used to remove the endothelial cell layer. The donor button is then grasped with toothed forceps in two locations, while Vannas scissors are used to trim the peripheral donor button (1 to 3 mm) from the endothelial side.

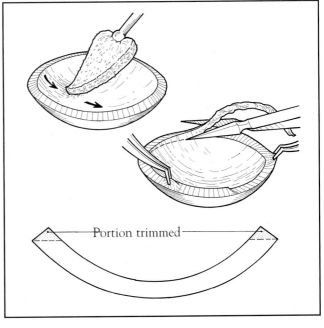

Portion trimmed

turn dark and simply contract. If the burned surface turns white, it indicates epithelial invasion. Lasering may also serve as a treatment, particularly in the early cases. Once the extent of epithelial downgrowth has been identified, involved iris tissue can be removed through a three-port vitrectomy approach. A straight transvitreal cryoprobe is then used to destruct the retrocorneal cells directly. The retrocorneal cells can sometimes be peeled in sheets using intraocular forceps. However, it is still necessary to freeze the bed to prevent recurrences.

Intracameral 5-FU application following the viscodissection of the membrane and peeling from the corneal endothelium was reported to be effective.

Always Remember...

In eyes with epithelial downgrowth confined to the cornea, transcorneal freezing with a regular cryoprobe may be sufficient, especially if the affected area is small. An intracameral air bubble is useful to provide an insulating effect and a more effective, controlled destruction. In more advanced cases, intracameral 5-FU can be applied.

Bibliography

Chiou AGY, Kaufman SC, Kaz K, Bauerman RW, Kaufman HE. Characterization of epithelial downgrowth by confocal microscopy. *J Cataract Refract Surg*. 1999;25:1172-1174.

Goodman DF, Gottsch JD. Lamellar corneal surgery. In: Gottsch JD, Stark WJ, Goldberg MF, eds. *Ophthalmic Surgery*. 5th ed. London: Arnold; 1999:131-137.

Goodman DF, Stark WJ, Gottsch JD. Corneal transplantation. In: Gottsch JD, Stark WJ, Goldberg MF, eds. *Ophthalmic Surgery*. 5th ed. London: 1999:119-130.

Matsuda M, Manabe R. The corneal endothelium following autokeratoplasty: a case report. *Acta Ophthalmol*. 1988;66:54-57.

Matsumoto Y, Dogru M, Goto E, et al. Autologous serum application in the treatment of neurotrophic keratopathy. *Ophthalmology*. 2004;111:1115-1120.

Murthy S, Bansal AK, Sridhar MS, Rao GN. Ipsilateral rotational autokeratoplasty: an alternative to penetrating keratoplasty in nonprogressive central corneal scars. *Cornea*. 2001;20:455-457.

Reed JW, Joyner SJ, Karuer WJ III. Penetrating keratoplasty for herpes zoster keratopathy. *Am J Ophthalmol*. 1989;107:257-261.

Rehany V, Waisman M. Suppression of corneal allograft rejection by systemic cyclosporine-A in heavily vascularized rabbit corneas following alkali burns. *Cornea*. 1994;13:447-453.

Sawa M, Tonishima T. The morphometry of the human corneal endothelium and follow-up of postoperative changes. *Jpn J Ophthalmol*. 1979;23:337-350.

Schimmelpfenning B, Baumgartner A. Einige manifestationen moglicher trophischer veraenderungen des corneaepithels nach herabgesetzten trigeminalfunktion. *Klin Monatsbl Augenheilkd*. 1988;192:149-153.

Shaikh AA, Damji KF, Mintsioulis G, et al. Bilateral epithelial downgrowth managed in one eye with intraocular 5-fluorouracil. *Arch Ophthalmol*. 2002;120:1396-1399.

Tanure MAG, Cohen EJ, Grewal S, Rapuano CJ, Laibson PR. Penetrating keratoplasty for Varicella-zoster virus keratopathy. *Cornea*. 2000;19:135-139.

Yagev R, Levy J, Sharer Z, Lifshitz T. Congenital insensitivity to pain with anhidrosis: ocular and systemic manifestations. *Am J Ophthalmol*. 1999;127:322-326.

CHAPTER 23

THREE
PEARLS TO MINIMIZE POSTKERATOPLASTY
ASTIGMATISM

Tushar Agarwal, MD; Namrata Sharma, MD; Rasik B.Vajpayee, MS, FRCSEd; and Samir A. Melki, MD, PhD

Despite numerous advances in corneal transplantation, post-penetrating keratoplasty astigmatism remains an important problem faced by the corneal surgeon. A range of 3 to 6 D of mean postkeratoplasty astigmatism is documented in various studies. Some of the factors responsible for the occurrence of high postkeratoplasty astigmatism are difficult to control. These include preexisting donor astigmatism and variability in individual healing responses. Other factors are related to surgical technique and may be helped by modifying the procedure using measures relating to graft centration, host trephination, and symmetric placement and tension of the corneal sutures (to ensure equal graft tissue distribution). This chapter describes other steps that may minimize the occurrence of high, as well as irregular, astigmatism after corneal transplantation.

PEARL #93: BETTER CHOICES IN GRAFT SIZE

The diameter and the shape of the corneal graft may influence the degree of postkeratoplasty astigmatism. Smaller diameter grafts are usually associated with higher degrees of astigmatism due to the proximity of the sutures to the visual axis. In situations of low endothelial cell counts, another disadvantage of small diameter grafts is the lower number of endothelial cells transplanted. Larger grafts induce less astigmatism but are at higher risk of rejection due to greater proximity to the limbal vasculature.

The disparity between the size of the graft and the host also has an influence over the astigmatic outcome after corneal transplantation. To reduce the amplitude of associated myopia, some surgeons advocate the use of a donor corneal button of a size similar to that of a host cut, especially for keratoconic corneas. However, tight suturing is sometimes required to achieve adequate wound apposition, possibly leading to higher degrees of postkeratoplasty astigmatism in these cases. The recommended disparity between a host cut and a donor graft either punched from the endothelial side or trephined from the epithelial side ranges between 0.25 to 0.5 mm, with the graft being larger in diameter. It is important to note that for grafts punched from the endothelial side, the button measures 0.2 mm less than the trephine used to cut it. The host bed diameter may vary in size if the cornea is too steep or too flat.

PEARL #94: AVOID OVAL TREPHINATION

An oval cut of the host cornea during the trephination would lead to the unequal or irregular disparity between the size of the host cut and the graft size. Such an event can cause problems in suturing and may ultimately result in severe post-penetrating keratoplasty astigmatism. The bridle traction sutures used to steady the eye may cause an oval cut if the force exerted by sutures holding the superior and inferior recti are transmitted to the cornea, causing elongation in a vertical direction. In these cases, corneal trephination leads to a horizontally oval host cut and subsequent astigmatic problems. However, traction sutures are necessary for corneal grafting surgery in deep-set eyes, narrow palpebral fissures, or in an eye that has rolled upward. Minimal traction, however, should be applied during trephination.

Similarly, application of a Flieringa ring can also transmit unequal traction forces to the host cornea, resulting in an oval cut (Figure 23-1). Use of Flieringa rings has been recommended in aphakic, pseudophakic, and pediatric eyes because the eyeball has a tendency to collapse in such eyes after the

Figure 23-1 (Pearl 94). Flieringa rings may exert excessive traction on the cornea, resulting in oval trephination and increased astigmatism.

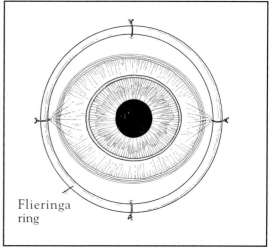

Flieringa
ring

trephination. Application of a Flieringa ring may prevent such a collapse. However, sutures applied to the sclera to fix the Flieringa ring may transmit unequal tension to the host cornea, leading to an irregular trephination (see Figure 23-1). Many surgeons do not use a Flieringa ring even if a globe collapse is a certainty after the trephination of host cornea. In such a situation, four full-thickness cardinal sutures are employed to initially secure the graft. Subsequently, the globe is reformed with the help of balanced salt solution, and the suturing is completed.

Similarly, tilting of the trephine or decentration of the Teflon block will produce an oval cut of the donor. A tilt of 20 degrees results in approximately 0.5 mm of disparity between the major and minor axis. Other factors that may distort the host or donor graft contour include a dull or damaged trephine, abnormally low or elevated IOP, and distortion of the globe from the lid speculum.

Always Remember...

> *Oval trephination of the host cornea may occur secondary to asymmetric torque on the cornea, tight bridle sutures, Flieringa rings, and inappropriate lid specula.*

PEARL #95: RUNNING VERSUS INTERRUPTED SUTURES

The technique of suturing a corneal graft to the host is an important variable affecting astigmatism after corneal transplantation. Surgeon's preference and experience, vascularity of the cornea, and age of the recipient influence the decision to use a running suture. A running suture offers the advantage of adjustment at 4 to 6 weeks to modify postkeratoplasty astigmatism. Single continuous suturing technique is associated with less final postoperative astigmatism compared with the interrupted suturing techniques because of even distribution provided by the single suture. Multiple interrupted sutures can disrupt the even distribution of corneal tension, thereby hindering astigmatism. Selective suture removal of interrupted sutures after the adequate healing of the host-graft junction can help in modifying postkeratoplasty astigmatism during the later stages of follow-up.

Running sutures can be applied using torque, antitorque, or no torque techniques, depending on the direction of intrastromal bite of the suture (Figures 23-2). After an evaluation of corneal topography, the sutures are adjusted if the amplitude of the astigmatism is >3.0 D. Using slit lamp biomicroscopy, suture adjustment is performed with tying forceps under topical anesthesia. The suture is rotated from the flatter meridian to the steeper meridian of the graft. It is preferable to use suture-tying forceps instead of jeweler's forceps to hold and pull the suture because the sharp edges of a jeweler's forceps can cut the suture.

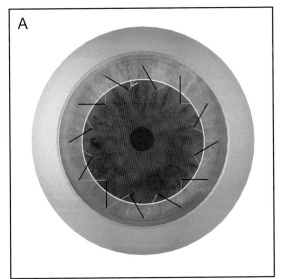

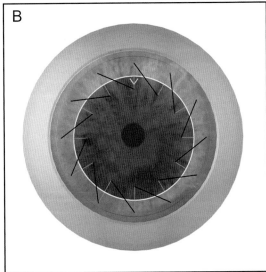

Figure 23-2 (Pearl 95). Running sutures with torque (A), antitorque (B), and no torque (C) techniques.

Surgical keratometers are useful for the assessment of corneal astigmatism induced at the time of surgery. Knowledge of the magnitude of astigmatism provides the surgeon with instant feedback about the effect of surgical maneuvers. In this regard, the Troutman keratometer is the most widely used intraoperative keratometer. Intraoperative suture adjustment permits more rapid visual rehabilitation, increased safety, and increased refractive stability.

The toricity of the graft and the suture can be readjusted, if needed, 3 to 5 days after the suture adjustment. Multiple suture adjustments of a running suture can be performed 4 to 6 weeks after the surgery.

Interrupted sutures are indicated in children and in patients with irregular and heavily vascularized host corneas. It is the suturing technique of choice for surgeons in their early stages of the learning curve. Sixteen interrupted sutures are normally used to suture a graft. During the early postoperative period, it is advisable to replace loose or tight interrupted sutures. During later stages, when the wound appears well healed, removing a tight suture can reduce the astigmatism.

Always Remember...

A running suture offers a better chance of modifying astigmatism because it may be adjusted by rotating the suture from the flatter meridian toward the steeper meridian.

BIBLIOGRAPHY

Bigar F, Herbort CP. Corneal transplantation. *Curr Opin Ophthalmol.* 1992;3(4):473-481.

Frangieh GT, Kwitko S, McDonnell PJ. Prospective corneal topographic analysis in surgery for postkeratoplasty astigmatism. *Arch Ophthalmol.* 1991;109(4):506-510.

Riddle HK Jr, Parker DA, Price FW Jr. Management of postkeratoplasty astigmatism. *Curr Opin Ophthalmol.* 1998;9(4):15-28.

Swinger CA. Postoperative astigmatism. *Surv Ophthalmol.* 1987;31(4):219-248.

Serdarevic ON, Renard GJ, Pouliquen Y. Randomized clinical trial of penetrating keratoplasty. Before and after suture removal comparison of intraoperative and postoperative suture adjustment. *Ophthalmology.* 1995;102(10):1497-503.

Vajpayee RB, Sharma V, Sharma N, Panda A, Taylor HR. Evaluation of techniques of single continuous suturing in penetrating keratoplasty. *Br J Ophthalmol.* 2001;85:134-138.

CHAPTER 24

THREE
PEARLS IN MANAGING POSTERIOR
VITREOUS PRESSURE DURING PENETRATING
KERATOPLASTY

Sadeer B. Hannush, MD

Penetrating keratoplasty is associated with a higher risk of complications than closed-eye anterior or posterior segment surgery. The open-sky hypotonus state is stressful for the eye and poses serious potential dangers. Adding to this stress is the general tendency of the vitreous body to push the iris-lens diaphragm anteriorly when the corneal button is off. In cases when corneal transplantation alone is being performed, the surgeon can usually control posterior pressure by simply constricting the pupil. If, on the other hand, keratoplasty is combined with surgery on the crystalline lens or management of a prosthetic lens implant in the setting of an intact posterior capsule, the surgical approach should be tailored accordingly.

PEARL #96: AVOID POSTERIOR VITREOUS PRESSURE: USING PHYSICS TO YOUR ADVANTAGE

When lens surgery, specifically cataract extraction, is combined with penetrating keratoplasty, consideration should be given to avoiding any external or internal forces that may increase pressure in the vitreous cavity. A lid speculum that does not contact the globe is ideal. The Jaffe lid speculum is well suited for this purpose. A scleral support ring may also be useful to avoid globe flaccidity. Furthermore, sutures around the ring that pull the globe slightly forward can help decrease internal pressure. Positioning the patient in a slight reverse Trendelenburg position and avoiding overextension of the neck may be helpful as well. The use of hyperosmotic agents such as Mannitol (Astra USA, Inc, Westboro, Mass) (eg, 50 cc of a 25% solution 30 minutes prior to the start of the procedure in adults) may allow the vitreous to shrink, thus diminishing the force it exerts on the iris-lens diaphragm. Finally, general anesthesia with muscle paralysis may be considered to allow for complete paralysis of the extraocular and lid muscles. A hypotensive technique, consisting of dropping the mean systemic blood pressure by approximately 30%, may be requested from the anesthesiologist.

Note: With the increasing popularity of laryngeal mask anesthesia (LMA), the ophthalmologist may not be aware that the patient is frequently not paralyzed in this setting. Communication between the eye surgeon and the anesthesiologist is of paramount importance. With LMA, if the patient is indeed not paralyzed, supplemental local anesthesia may be offered to paralyze the extraocular muscles.

Always Remember…

Avoid excessive periocular anesthesia to reduce intraconal and vitreous pressure.

PEARL #97: CLOSED-CHAMBER OR OPEN-SKY PHACO-ASSISTED CATARACT EXTRACTION

If the corneal pathology allows visualization of the lens, cataract surgery may be performed as usual through a clear corneal incision, a scleral tunnel, or even a partial corneal trephination wound. However, in the case of the latter, the phacoemulsification needle may cause too much distortion of the wound to allow visualization of the lens. In the setting of corneal edema, the epithelium may be removed, a technique vitreoretinal surgeons frequently employed in the past. Because the surgery is performed under a dome of viscoelastic, any posterior pressure is balanced until after the IOL implant insertion and constriction of the pupil. The surgeon may proceed with the graft at this point.

Figure 24-1 (Pearl 97). After phaco-assisted open-sky cataract extraction, the IOL is placed inside the capsular bag, thus stabilizing the iris-lens diaphragm.

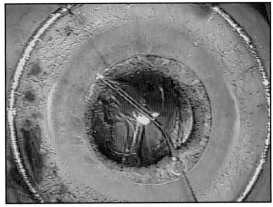

Figure 24-2 (Pearl 97). With the IOL inside the capsular bag, the pupil is easily constricted pharmacologically.

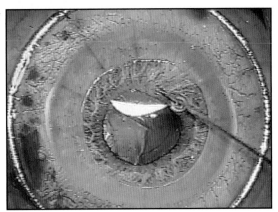

Many problems with open-sky cataract extraction are secondary to radial dissection of the can-opener or rhexis capsulotomy tear due to the forward force exerted by the vitreous, resulting in posterior extension of a radial tear and vitreous loss. This can be minimized by performing a small rhexis (4 to 5 mm) during which a second instrument (such as a cyclodialysis spatula) is used to push the lens nucleus down. Because the opening will not allow expression of the lens nucleus, phacoemulsification may be used to divide the lens into two or four fragments, which are then removed by high-vacuum aspiration. After cortical clean up, a foldable or one-piece PMMA implant may be placed inside the capsular bag to stabilize the iris-capsule diaphragm, allowing constriction of the pupil and placement of the donor button (Figures 24-1 and 24-2).

Always Remember...

In the case of a cataract with adequate visualization through the cloudy cornea, lens extraction may be performed with greater safety prior to removal of the corneal button than through an open-sky approach.

Placing an implant inside the capsular bag with a small capsulorrhexis allows the use of the bag diaphragm to control posterior vitreous pressure.

PEARL #98: VITRECTOMY IN KERATOPLASTY

There are instances when all efforts fail to control posterior pressure before penetrating keratoplasty, during the procedure, or at the end while trying to reform the anterior chamber. The cornea may be too cloudy to allow for a closed-chamber approach to the lens. An example is a short eye (<21 mm

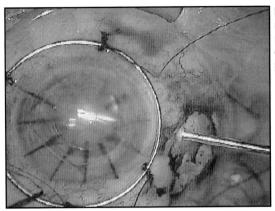

Figure 24-3 (Pearl 98). Shortly after trephination, posterior pressure is encountered not responsive to anterior management techniques. A limited pars plana vitrectomy decompresses the vitreous, allowing completion of the procedure.

axial length) with a very cloudy cornea and shallow chamber after a bout of angle-closure glaucoma or chronic inflammation. Decompressing the vitreous may prove very useful in allowing surgery on the lens and/or reformation of the anterior chamber at the end of the case. A conjunctivotomy is placed 3.5 mm posterior to the limbus, usually in the superotemporal quadrant. Using an MVR blade, a sclerotomy is then performed at that location followed by the introduction of a vitrectomy instrument (Figure 24-3). In general, peristaltic pumps (certain phacoemulsification units) should be avoided. The settings are usually for a cutting speed >600 cuts per minute and vacuum of 100 to 150 mm Hg. A few seconds of cutting and aspiration with the vitrectomy tip well within view through the pupil is usually more than adequate to allow for decompression of the vitreous cavity and successful completion of the procedure. The sclerotomy site is then closed with absorbable sutures. This technique has been very rewarding in managing severe posterior pressure. With the advent of 25-gauge vitrectomy technology, the vitreous decompression may be performed through a small suteless sclerotomy.

Always Remember…

Do not hesitate to perform a limited pars plana vitrectomy to decompress the eye during open-sky anterior segment surgery.

Consider preparing the sclera and having the vitrectomy machine setup in high-risk cases and/or in monocular patients.

BIBLIOGRAPHY

Barraquer J, Rutllán J. Intraoperative complications of penetrating keratoplasty. In: *Atlas de Microcirugía de la Córnea. Barcelona:* la Ed Scriba; 1982:325-328.

Brightbill T, Frederick K. Adult penetrating keratoplasty. In: *Corneal Surgery: Theory, Technique and Tissue.* St. Louis, Mo: CV Mosby; 1993:210.

Krupin T, Kolker A. Keratoplasty: managing the vitreous. In: *Atlas of Complications in Ophthalmic Surgery.* St. Louis, Mo: Wolfe/ Mosby; 1993:5-7.

Rao SK, Padmanabhan P. Combined phacoemulsification and penetrating keratoplasty. *Ophthalmic Surg Lasers.* 1991;30(6):488-491.

Shimada H, Nakashizuka H, Mori R, Mizutani Y. Expanded indications for 25-gauge transconjunctival vitrectomy. *Jpn J Ophthalmol.* 2005;49(5):397-401.

Shimomura Y, Hosotani H, Kiritoshi A, Watanabe H, Tano Y. Core vitrectomy preceding triple corneal procedures in patients at high risk for increased posterior chamber pressure. *Jpn J Ophthalmol.* 1997;41(4):251-254.

Sridhar MS, Murthy S, Bansal AK, Rao GN. Corneal triple procedure: indications, complications, and outcomes: a developing country scenario. *Cornea.* 2000;19(3):333-335.

Tei M, Shimamoto, Yasuhara T, Komori H, Oda H, Kinoshita S. A new non-trocar system for 25 gauge transconjunctival pars plana vitrectomy. *Am J Ophthalmol.* 2005;139(6):1130-1133.

CHAPTER 25

THREE
PEARLS IN POSTERIOR KERATOPLASTY

Tae-Young Chung, MD and Dimitri T. Azar, MD

Penetrating keratoplasty is currently the surgical method of choice in corneal endothelial diseases such as Fuchs dystrophy and aphakic and pseudophakic bullous keratopathy. However, selective transplantation of only the diseased posterior corneal tissue (endothelium, DM, and posterior stroma) is an attractive alternative. This procedure, termed posterior keratoplasty, has several theoretical advantages over penetrating keratoplasty. These include faster visual recovery, less postoperative astigmatism, and lower risk of intraoperative complications and wound dehiscence. In this chapter, we discuss the current techniques of posterior keratoplasty.

PEARL #99: FEMTOSECOND LASER-ASSISTED SMALL INCISION DEEP LAMELLAR ENDOTHELIAL KERATOPLASTY

The technique of endothelial replacement through a superior scleral pocket wound was first described by Gerrit Melles and termed posterior lamellar keratoplasty (PLK). The technique and instrumentation was modified by Mark Terry and Paula Ousley and termed deep lamellar endothelial keratoplasty (DLEK). Recently, this original DLEK technique was modified to small incision DLEK in an attempt to reduce postoperative astigmatism and, thereby, result in better visual outcome. However, manual lamellar dissection is not only time consuming and technically difficult but may also result in corneal perforation and interface scarring.

Recent progress has led us to use the femtosecond (10^{-15} seconds) laser in creating the LASIK flap. The femtosecond laser demonstrated improved uniformity of the flap and better predictability of the flap thickness than mechanical microkeratomes. Here we will describe the basic techniques of femtosecond laser-assisted small incision DLEK for treating patients with corneal endothelial dysfunction.

The surgical procedure is performed under topical anesthesia. The donor corneoscleral button is mounted in a dedicated artificial anterior chamber. Ultrasound pachymetry is performed prior to donor lamellar dissection. This is to make sure that the donor corneal thickness is between 500 and 550 μm in order to approximate the graft thickness of 100 to 150 μm. Then, the femtosecond laser is used to create a corneal flap of 9.5-mm diameter and 400-mm thickness. After laser application, stromal and side cut adhesions are fully released and the anterior corneal flap is fully lifted. This previously prepared donor corneoscleral button is then placed in the medium and transported to the operating room. An 8.0-mm epithelial marking is made in the recipient cornea prior to a 5.0-mm scleral incision, and a deep lamellar pocket is created down to about 75% to 85% corneal thickness over the entire cornea. The posterior recipient disc is then excised with Cindy scissors (Bausch & Lomb, St. Louis, Mo) using the 8.0-mm epithelial mark as a template. The excised posterior recipient disc is removed from the lamellar pocket and spread out over the recipient corneal epithelium to verify the size. Viscoelastic is then removed from the anterior chamber using standard irrigation-aspiration techniques. Complete removal of viscoelasctic is required for later graft self-attachment. The anterior flap of the prepared donor corneoscleral button is excised using scissors, and the posterior part is punched out with an 8.0-mm trephine (Katena, Danville, NJ). This 8.0-mm posterior donor disc is then folded endothelial side inside with a layer of viscoelastic (Healon [Pharmacia, Peapack, NJ]) coating the endothelium and inserted into the anterior

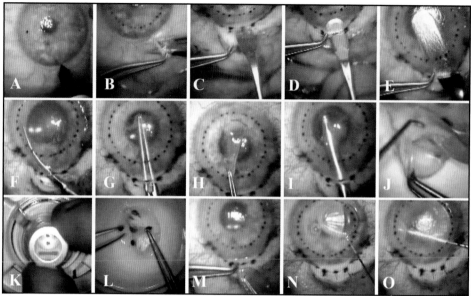

Figure 25-1 (Pearl 99). Intraoperative image of femtosecond laser-assisted small incision DLEK. (A) An 8.0-mm ink mark is made on the epithelial surface. (B) Conjunctival peritomy is made. (C) A 5.0-mm superior scleral tunnel incision is made. (D) A deep lamellar pocket is created with a crescent blade. (E) Further dissection is made over the entire cornea using a straight Devers dissector (Bausch & Lomb, St. Louis, MO) and a curved Devers dissector. (F) Posterior recipient disc is excised using scissors. (G) Posterior recipient disc is removed from the anterior chamber. (H) Posterior recipient disc is spread out over the recipient corneal epithelium in order to verify the size. (I) Viscoelastic is completely removed using irrigation-aspiration techniques. (J) The anterior corneal flap is removed from the posterior part of the prepared donor corneoscleral button, which was dissected using a femtosecond laser at 400 µm in depth. (K) The posterior donor button is placed on a Teflon block with the endothelial-side up, and a trephine is used to punch out the posterior donor disc. (L) The posterior donor disc is then folded endothelial-side inside with a layer of viscoelastic coating the endothelium. (M) Folded posterior donor disc is inserted into the anterior chamber with forceps through the small incision. (N) An air bubble is injected underneath the graft to place the donor stromal surface into contact with the recipient stromal bed for self-adhesion. (O) Graft position is adjusted with a Sinskey hook.

chamber through the small incision using forceps. The folded donor disc is opened and attached to the recipient stromal bed by injecting an air bubble underneath the graft. The graft position is adjusted using Sinskey hook to make sure that the donor edges are tucked anterior to the recipient bed edges to prevent later graft dislocation. The scleral wound is closed with 2 or 3 interrupted 10-0 nylon sutures, and air is replaced with balanced salt solution to normalize the IOP.

Always Remember...

Be sure to completely remove the viscoelastic from the anterior chamber and the pocket after removing the posterior recipient disc.

Make sure that the donor edges are tucked anterior to the recipient bed edges to prevent later dislodgement of the donor disc.

PEARL #100: DESCEMET'S STRIPPING AND TRANSPLANTATION OF ENDOTHELIUM (MELLES AND PRICE TECHNIQUES)

Since the stroma is usually not affected in corneas with endothelial dysfunction, one way of treating corneal endothelial disease may be to replace only the endothelial cells. A surgical technique for

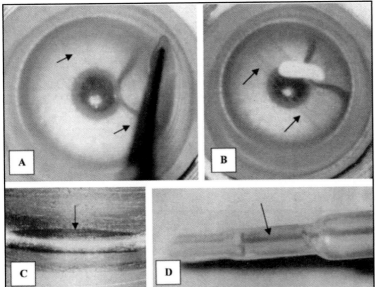

Figure 25-2A (Pearl 100). Preparation of donor DM. (A) After partial trephination of the posterior side of a corneoscleral button, a circular portion of DM (arrows) is stripped from the button with fine forceps. (B) After complete detachment, a Descemet roll (arrows) forms spontaneously, with the endothelium on the outside. (C) To better visualize the donor tissue, the donor DM is stained with trypan blue. (D) The Descemet roll (arrow) is then sucked into an injector. (Reprinted from Melles GR, Lander F, Rietveld FJ. Transplantation of DM carrying viable endothelium through a small scleral incision. *Cornea.* 2002;21(4):415-418.)

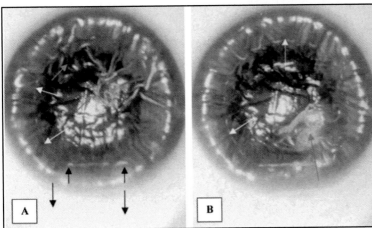

Figure 25-2B (Pearl 100). Intraoperative pictures of the recipient eye. (A) After filling the anterior chamber with air, through a scleral incision (black arrows), a descemetorhexis is performed (white arrows). (B) The descemetorhexis has been completed over 360 degrees, and the excised membrane is visible on top of the cornea (red arrow). (Reprinted from Melles GR, Lander F, Rietveld FJ. Transplantation of DM carrying viable endothelium through a small scleral incision. *Cornea.* 2002;21(4):415-418.)

transplantation of the endothelium, with the use of its DM as a carrier, was recently described by Gerrit Melles. With this procedure, less interface haze and less operation time is expected. Here, we will describe the surgical procedures.

For the Melles technique, the donor corneoscleral button is mounted endothelial side up on a custom-made holder with a suction cup, and the holder carrying the button is completely immersed in balanced salt solution. After superficial trephination of in the posterior stroma with a 9.0-mm trephine (Ophtec, Groningen, The Netherlands), a circular portion of DM is stripped from the posterior stroma using fine forceps. The stripped DM forms a Descemet roll after completion of detachment, and a 9.0-mm diameter flap of posterior DM with the endothelium at the outer side is obtained. The Descemet roll is stained with 0.06% trypan blue (VisionBlue [DORC International, Zuidland, The Netherlands]) to better visualize the donor tissue and is sucked into a custom-made injector.

A 5.0-mm sclerocorneal tunnel incision is made in the recipient eye at the 12 o'clock position. Then, the anterior chamber is completely filled with air to create an optical interface at the corneal endothelial surface. A 9.0-mm mark is made on the corneal epithelium to outline the size of the DM that is to be removed. With a custom-made scraper (DORC International), DM is then carefully stripped off the posterior stroma by loosening the membrane at the 6 o'clock position and pulling it toward the incision

Figure 25-2C (Pearl 100). Intraoperative pictures of the implantation of the donor DM in the recipient eye. (A) Through the scleral tunnel incision (black arrows), the donor DM (white arrow) is brought into the anterior chamber with the injector. (B) The Descemet roll (green arrow) is positioned along the vertical meridian of the eye. (C) By injection of balanced salt solution onto the anterior side of the donor DM tissue, the membrane (green arrow) is unfolded and spread out over the iris. (D) With a blunt canula, air is then injected underneath the donor DM, to position the membrane (green arrow) against the recipient posterior corneal stroma. (Reprinted from Melles GR, Lander F, Rietveld FJ. Transplantation of DM carrying viable endothelium through a small scleral incision. *Cornea.* 2002;21(3):415-418.)

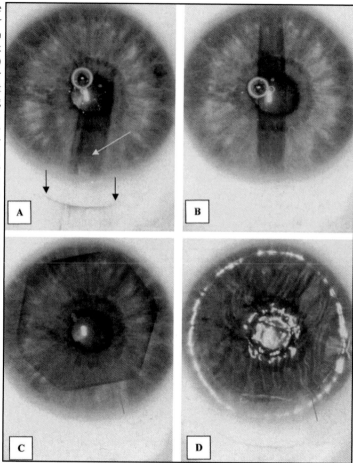

at 12 o'clock. Once the leading edge is created at the 6 o'clock position, the remainder of the membrane can be stripped off from the recipient posterior stroma with forceps similar to the capsulorhexis. After a complete 9.0-mm diameter Descemetorhexis, the membrane is removed from the eye.

For the Price DSAEK (descemet stripping automated endothelial keratoplasty) technique, a posterior stromal layer with endothelium is transplanted as in the DLEK technique. For the Melles technique, the donor Descemet roll is brought into the anterior chamber and oriented along the vertical meridian of the recipient eye. By gently manipulating the inner portion of the Descemet roll with a canula and injecting balanced salt solution onto the anterior side of the donor DM, the membrane is unfolded and spread out over the iris. The canula is then used to inject an air bubble underneath the donor DM to position the membrane against the recipient posterior stroma. If necessary, the donor tissue is repositioned by pulling the edge of the transplant with fine forceps.

Always Remember...

After completion of Descemetorhexis, the Descemet roll forms with the endothelium at the outer side.

Pearl# 101: Microkeratome-Assisted Posterior Keratoplasty

A significant problem of lamellar keratoplasty using manual dissection may be the postoperative interface opacity caused by stromal scarring. One of the merits of microkeratome dissection over manual

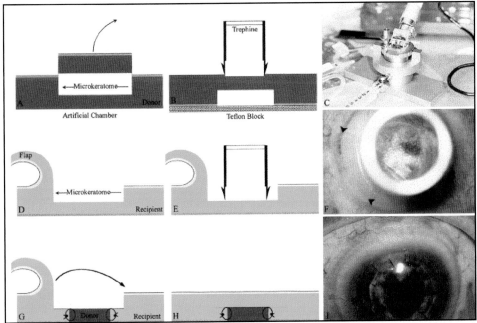

Figure 25-3 (Pearl 101). (A) A donor lenticule is excised using a microkeratome and a dedicated artificial anterior chamber and discarded. (B) The donor cornea is placed endothelial-side up on a Teflon block, and a trephine is used to punch a donor stromal button (red). (C) The microkeratome is engaged in a dedicated anterior chamber to prepare the donor lenticule. (D) A hinged anterior stromal flap is created in the host cornea using a microkeratome and lifted. (E) A trephine is used to excise the posterior host stroma and endothelium. (F) An intraoperative photograph shows the host anterior cornea after the microkeratome cut and flap lifting (arrowhead), illustrating the application of the trephine. (G) The donor stromal button (red) is transplanted onto the host bed (green) and secured using sutures (black). (H) The host corneal flap is refloated over the transplanted donor button. (I) A postoperative photograph of a patient treated with MAPK shows posterior stromal sutures under the flap. (Reprinted from Azar DT, Jain S, Samburusky R, Strauss L. Microkeratome-assisted posterior keratoplasty. *J Cataract Refract Surg.* 2001;27(3):353-356.)

dissection is that we can reduce the postoperative interface opacity, since the interface scarring is almost absent after microkeratome dissection in LASIK. Moreover, the flap can be lifted for excimer laser PRK treatment over posterior button to correct residual refractive errors. Here we will describe the surgical procedures of microkeratome-assisted posterior keratoplasty (MAPK).

An artificial anterior chamber is used to prepare the donor stromal button. A microkeratome (automated corneal shaper or Hansatome [Bausch & Lomb, St. Louis, Mo]) creates an 8.5- to 9.5-mm diameter, 180-μm thick anterior corneal cap without a hinge, and it is discarded. The donor cornea is then placed on a Teflon block with the endothelial side up, and a 6.0- to 8.0-mm trephine is used to punch the donor stromal button.

The recipient's cornea is marked with sterile skin marker or gentian violet to allow for precise reposition of the anterior corneal flap. A hinged anterior corneal flap 8.5 to 9.5 mm in diameter and 180 μm in thickness is created using a microkeratome. The suction ring is centered on the recipient's cornea over the pupil. The suction is activated and IOP is checked to be 80 mm Hg. The hinged anterior corneal flap is created and elevated using a flat spatula. A 6.0- to 8.0-mm trephine is used to perform a full-thickness trephination to excise the posterior stroma, DM, and endothelium of the recipient central cornea. Viscoelastic is placed into the anterior chamber. The donor stromal button is placed onto the recipient bed and secured using interrupted nonabsorbable 10-0 nylon sutures. The hinged anterior corneal flap is refloated over the donor stromal button and allowed to seal into place. Sutures or bandage contact lens may be used to secure the corneal flap.

Always Remember…

If the swelling of donor cornea is not reversed before the donor button preparation, a thinner-than-intended donor cornea may result postoperatively.

Bibliography

Azar DT, Jain S, Sambursky R. Microkeratome-assisted posterior keratoplasty. *J Cataract Refract Surg.* 2001;27:353-356.

Azar DT, Jain S, Sambursky R. A new surgical technique of microkeratome-assisted deep lamellar keratoplasty with a hinged flap. *Arch Ophthalmol.* 2000;118:1112-1115.

Melles GR, Lander F, Rietveld FJ. Transplantation of Descemet's membrane carrying viable endothelium through a small scleral incision. *Cornea.* 2002;21:415-418.

Melles GR, Wijdh RH, Nieuwendaal CP. A technique to excise the Descemet membrane from a recipient cornea (Descemetorhexis). *Cornea.* 2004;23:286-288.

Price FW Jr, Price MO. Descemet's stripping with endothelial keratoplasty in 50 eyes: a refractive neutral corneal transplant. *J Refract Surg.* 2005;21:339-345.

Terry MA, Ousley PJ. Deep lamellar endothelial keratoplasty in the first United States patients: early clinical results. *Cornea.* 2001;20:239-243.

Terry MA, Ousley PJ. Small-incision deep lamellar endothelial keratoplasty (DLEK): six-month results in the first prospective clinical study. *Cornea.* 2005;24:59-65.

Terry MA, Ousley PJ, Will B. A practical femtosecond laser procedure for DLEK endothelial transplantation: cadaver eye histology and topography. *Cornea.* 2005;24:453-459.

INDEX